Clinical Cases in Neurology

D1615498

Edited by

AHV Schapira

Chairman, University Department of Clinical Neurosciences
Royal Free and University College Medical School
and Institute of Neurology, University College London,
London, UK

and

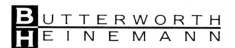

LP Rowland

Professor of Neurology, Department of Neurology
Columbia University College of Physicians & Surgeons,
Neurological Institute,
Columbia-Presbyterian Medical Center,
New York, USA

BUTTERWORTH
HEINEMANN

OXFORD AUCKLAND BOSTON JOHANNESBURG MELBOURNE NEW DELHI

Butterworth-Heinemann Linacre House, Jordan Hill, Oxford OX2 8DP
225 Wildwood Avenue, Woburn, MA 01801-2041
A division of Reed Educational and Professional Publishing Ltd

ℛ A member of the Reed Elsevier plc group

First published 2001

British Library Cataloguing in Publication Data
Clinical cases in neurology
 1. Neurology – Case studies   2. Nervous system – Diseases –
Diagnosis – Case studies
 I. Schapira, A.H.V.   II. Rowland, Lewis P.
 616.8

Library of Congress Cataloguing in Publication Data
Clinical cases in neurology/edited by A.H.V. Schapira and L.P. Rowland.
  p.;cm
  Includes index
  ISBN 0 7506 4304 8
  1. Nervous system–Diseases–Case studies. I. Schapira, Antony H.V.
  (Anthony Henry Vernon) II. Rowland, Lewis P.
  [DNLM: 1. Nervous System Diseases–Case Report. WL 140 C63995 2001]
  RC359 .C56
  616.8′049–dc21   00-068888

 ISBN 0 7506 4304 8

Typeset by David Gregson Associates
Printed and bound in Great Britain by MPG, Bodmin, Cornwall

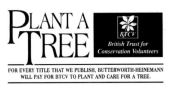

PLANT A TREE
British Trust for
Conservation Volunteers
FOR EVERY TITLE THAT WE PUBLISH, BUTTERWORTH-HEINEMANN
WILL PAY FOR BTCV TO PLANT AND CARE FOR A TREE.

Contents

Abbreviations

ADEM	acute disseminated encephalomyelitis
ADHD	attention deficit hyperactivity disorder
AIDS	acquired immunodeficiency syndrome
ALS	amyotrophic lateral sclerosis
ALS-PUMNS	amyotrophic lateral sclerosis with probable upper motor neuron signs
AMAN	acute motor axonal neuropathy
ANA	antinuclear antibodies
ANCA	antineutrophil cytoplasmic autoantibodies
BSE	bovine spongiform encephalopathy
CADASIL	cerebral autosomal dominant arteriopathy with subcortical infarcts and leukoencephalopathy
CIDP	chronic inflammatory demyelinating polyneuropathy
CJD	Creutzfeldt–Jakob disease
CSF	cerebrospinal fluid
CT	chemotherapy
DNA	deoxyribonucleic acid
FHM	familial hemiplegic migraine
FSHD	facioscapulohumeral dystrophy
h-IBM	hereditary inclusion body myositis
HIV	human immunodeficiency virus
HMSN	hereditary motor and sensory neuropathy
HNPP	hereditary neuropathy with liability to pressure palsies
HZV	herpes zoster virus
IBM	inclusion body myositis
IVIG	intravenous immunoglobulin
JME	juvenile myoclonic epilepsy
LGMD	limb girdle muscular dystrophies
MELAS	mitochondrial encephalomyopathy with lactic acidosis and stroke-like episodes
MJD	Machado–Joseph disease
MN	motor neuropathy
MND	motor neuron disease
MRI	magnetic resonance imaging
MRS	magnetic resonance spectroscopy

NCSE	non-convulsive status epilepticus
NMS	neuroleptic malignant syndrome
OCB	obsessive-compulsive behavior
PANDAS	pediatric autoimmune neuropsychiatric disorders associated with streptococcal infection
PCNSL	primary central nervous system lymphoma
PML	progressive multifocal leukoencephalopathy
PSMA	progressive spinal muscular atrophy
RNA	ribonucleic acid
SMA	spinal muscular atrophy
SNAP	sensory nerve action potential
XSBMA	X-linked spinobulbar muscular atrophy

List of Contributors

John C. M. Brust, MD
Professor of Clinical Neurology, Columbia University College of Physicians & Surgeons (Director, Department of Neurology, Harlem Hospital Center, New York, NY 10037), Neurological Institute, Columbia-Presbyterian Medical Center, New York, NY 10032, US

Lisa M. DeAngelis, MD
Chairman, Department of Neurology, Memorial Sloan-Kettering Cancer Center, New York, NY 10021, USA

Valsamma Eapen, MBBS, DPM, MRCPsych., PhD
Associate Professor in Child Psychiatry, Faculty of Medicine, UAE University, UAE; Honorary Lecturer, Royal Free & University College Medical School, University College London, London W1N 8AA, UK

Stanley Fahn, MD
H. Houston Merritt Professor of Neurology, Department of Neurology, Columbia University College of Physicians & Surgeons, Neurological Institute, Columbia-Presbyterian Medical Center, New York, NY 10032, USA

Hassan Fathallah-Shaykh, MD
Head, Section of Neuro-Oncology, Assistant Professor, Rush University Medical Center, Department of Neurology, Columbia University College of Physicians & Surgeons, Neurological Institute, Columbia-Presbyterian Medical Center, New York, NY 10032, USA

Steven J. Frucht, MD
Assistant Professor of Neurology, Department of Neurology, Columbia University College of Physicians & Surgeons, Neurological Institute, Columbia-Presbyterian Medical Center, New York, NY 10032, USA

Lionel Ginsberg, BSc, MB, BS, PhD, FRCP
Consultant Neurologist, Royal Free Hospital, London NW3 2QG, UK

Arthur P. Hays, MD
Associate Professor of Pathology, Department of Pathology, Columbia University College of Physicians & Surgeons, Columbia-Presbyterian Medical Center, New York, NY 10032, USA

Susan T. Iannaccone, MD
Director, Neuromuscular Disease & Neurorehabilitation, Texas Scottish Ritu Hospital for Children; Professor of Neurology, University of Texas Southwestern Medical Center, Dallas, TX 75219, USA

Christopher Kennard, PhD, FRCP
Professor of Clinical Neurology, Head Division of Neuroscience & Psychological Medicine, Imperial College School of Medicine, London W6 8RP, UK

Dora Leung, MD
Assistant Professor of Clinical Neurology (Harlem Hospital Center, New York, NY 10037), Columbia University College of Physicians & Surgeons, Neurological Institute, Columbia-Presbyterian Medical Center, New York, NY 10032, USA

Karen S. Marder, MD
Associate Professor of Neurology (Sergievsky Center & in The Taub Institute), Department of Neurology, Columbia University College of Physicians & Surgeons, Neurological Institute, Columbia-Presbyterian Medical Center, New York, NY 10032, USA

Anil Mendiratta, MD
Clinical Fellow in Neurology, Department of Neurology (Comprehensive Epilepsy Center/EEG), Columbia University College of Physicians & Surgeons, Neurological Institute, Columbia-Presbyterian Medical Center, New York, NY 10032, USA

Dominic J. Mort, BA, MRCP
Clinical Research Fellow, Imperial College School of Medicine, London W6 8RP, UK

Richard W. Orrell BSc, MD, MRCP
Senior Lecturer and Consultant Neurologist, University Department of Clinical Neurosciences, Royal Free & University College Medical School & Institute of Neurology, University College London, London NW3 2PF, UK

Richard A. Prayson, MD
Department of Anatomic Pathology, Cleveland Clinic Foundation, Cleveland OH 44195, USA

Timothy A. Pedley, MD
Henry & Lucy Moses Professor & Chairman, Department of Neurology, Columbia University College of Physicians & Surgeons, Neurological Institute, Columbia-Presbyterian Medical Center, New York, NY 10032, USA

Jeffrey J. Raizer, MD
Clinical Assistant, Department of Neurology, Memorial Sloan-Kettering Cancer Center, New York NY 10021, USA

Mary M. Robertson MBChB, MD, DPM, FRCPsych
Professor of Neuropsychiatry, Department of Psychiatry, The National Hospital for Neurology & Neurosurgery, University College London, London W1N 8AA, UK

Roger N. Rosenberg, MD
Department of Neurology, University of Texas Southwestern Medical Center, Dallas TX 75219, USA

Lewis P. Rowland, MD
Professor of Neurology, Department of Neurology, Columbia University College of Physicians & Surgeons, Neurological Institute, Columbia-Presbyterian Medical Center, New York, NY 10032, USA

Todd D. Rozen, MD
Assistant Professor of Neurology/Headache Specialist, Jefferson Headache Center, Thomas Jefferson University Hospital, Philadelphia PA 19107, USA

Richard A. Rudick, MD
Hazel Prior Hostetler Professor of Neurology; Director, Mellen Center for Multiple Sclerosis Treatment & Research, Cleveland Clinic Foundation, Cleveland OH 44195, USA

Anthony H.V. Schapira, DSc, MD, FRCP, FMedSci
Chairman, University Department of Clinical Neurosciences, Royal Free & University College Medical School & Institute of Neurology, University College London, London NW3 2PF, UK

Stephen D. Silberstein, MD, FACP
Professor of Neurology, Jefferson Headache Center, Thomas Jefferson Universityospital, Hospital, Philadelphia PA 19107, USA

Anchi Wang, MD
Department of Neurology, University of Texas Southwestern Medical Center, Dallas TX 75219, USA

William B. Young, M.D.
Assistant Professor of Neurology, Thomas Jefferson University Hospital, Philadelphia PA 19107, USA

Preface

The past decade has brought enormous advances to the basic and clinical neurosciences. Neuroimaging and molecular genetics have transformed clinical practice. Nevertheless, neurology is still a quintessentially clinical discipline, generating a diagnosis from the history and physical signs, then using appropriate laboratory tests for confirmation. The neurology field is replete with large multi-volume texts that cover the broad spectrum of neurological disorders. However, discussion of clinical cases has long been an integral part of neurological training, education and enjoyment. We have therefore collected a series of case histories that are both challenging and informative, combining each with a discussion of the differential diagnosis and an up to date review of relevant material. We have endeavoured to ensure consistency of presentation throughout the book but neurological problems do not all fit neatly into the same format and so we have been flexible with this approach. We have sought to include a cross section of neurological disorders in this book but naturally the list is not exhaustive. Most of all we have attempted to produce a book that will be useful and also enjoyable to read. Each case is first described as a diagnostic problem. The discussion ends with the mention of a defining laboratory test or postmortem examination that settles the diagnosis. References are given separately at the end of each chapter. We are grateful to all the contributing authors who worked hard in crafting their cases. We should also like to thank Melanie Tait, Zoë Youd and Kieran Price for all their support and effort in producing the book.

A.H.V. Schapira
Lewis P. Rowland

Acute neuropathies

Clinical history and examination

A 63-year-old, right-handed woman was admitted to the hospital because of progressive limb muscle weakness and sensory disturbance.

Six weeks previously she had abruptly developed pain in her right calf and suffered several falls because of a right foot-drop. Three weeks later she noticed numbness of the thumb, index and middle fingers of the right hand with weakness and loss of dexterity. Numbness of the left little finger subsequently became apparent. On the day of admission she became unable to walk because of the sudden development of severe weakness of the left leg, the weakness of the right foot having persisted. There was no history of sphincter disturbance and no neck or back pain. The pain in the right calf had improved.

She had been well until 2 years before the onset of the neurological symptoms. At that time, her right eye had become painful and red. She was seen at another hospital and prescribed topical corticosteroids with benefit. Six months later, her hearing deteriorated over the course of a few weeks. Investigations at a third hospital showed a mixed pattern of conductive and sensorineural hearing loss, worse on the left. Bilateral middle ear effusions were detected on examination. Grommets were inserted without improvement.

There was no family history of neuromuscular disease. She was a non-smoker and drank little alcohol. She had had no exposure to trauma or toxic materials and had not traveled abroad. During the year before her neurological illness she had lost her appetite and 7 kg in weight. She was not taking any regular medication.

The temperature was 36.7°C, the pulse was 80 per minute and the respirations were 14 per minute. The blood pressure was 140/90 mmHg.

On neurological examination, cognitive function and speech were normal. Fundoscopy showed normal appearances of the optic discs. The remainder of the cranial nerve examination was also normal, with the

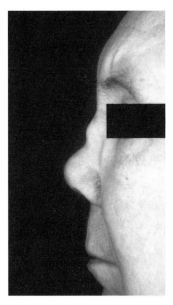

Fig. 1.1. Patient's facial appearance in profile, showing 'saddle nose' deformity.

exception of a sensorineural pattern of hearing loss, worse on the left, on tuning fork tests. Examination of the limbs showed wasting of the antero-lateral muscle compartment of the right leg. There was weakness of the distal right upper limb predominantly involving flexor pollicis longus, flexor indicis, abductor pollicis brevis and opponens pollicis (all MRC grade 2/5). In the right leg, there was weakness of ankle dorsiflexion and eversion (both 1/5) and extensor hallucis longus (0/5). There was more profound and widespread weakness of the left leg, involving all movements of the ankle and toes (0/5). Tendon reflexes were normal in the upper limbs and at the knees. Both ankle reflexes were absent, as were the plantar responses. Sensory testing revealed impaired position and vibration sensation in the feet. Cutaneous sensation of light touch and pinprick was reduced in the right thumb, index and middle fingers, left little finger, and both legs in a stocking distribution below the knees. She was unable to walk unaided. Examination of the cardiovascular and respiratory systems and the abdomen was normal. The only other finding on general examination was the presence of a 'saddle nose' deformity (Fig. 1.1). Review of family photographs indicated that this deformity had been acquired within the previous 5–10 years.

Routine hematological and biochemical investigations yielded a number of abnormalities (Table 1.1). The dominant findings were a normochromic, normocytic anemia with grossly elevated erythrocyte sedimentation rate and C-reactive protein, and deranged liver function tests. Though serum

Table 1.1. Results of blood tests.*

Variable (unit)	Value	Normal range
Hemoglobin (g/dl)	9.8	11.5–15.5
Hematocrit	0.32	0.35–0.47
Mean corpuscular volume (fl)	91	80–100
Platelets ($\times 10^9$/l)	435	140–400
Leukocytes ($\times 10^9$/l)	11.8	3.7–9.5
Neutrophils ($\times 10^9$/l)	8.9	1.7–7.5
Erythrocyte sedimentation rate (mm/h)	105	0–20
Urea (mmol/l)	7.0	3.0–6.5
Potassium (mmol/l)	4.3	3.5–5.0
Sodium (mmol/l)	134	135–145
Creatinine (μmol/l)	135	60–120
Albumin (g/l)	27	35–50
Total bilirubin (μmol/l)	6	5–17
Alkaline phosphatase (u/l)	260	<130
Alanine aminotransferase (u/l)	57	<40
Aspartate aminotransferase (u/l)	68	<40
Glucose (mmol/l)	5.3	2.9–5.3
C-reactive protein (mg/l)	48	<5

*The results of other routine tests were normal.

urea and creatinine were normal or near-normal, creatinine clearance was low at 67 ml/min. Thyroid function, syphilis serology and serum vitamin B12 and folate were all normal or negative. Serum immunoglobulins were within the normal range and protein electrophoresis showed no evidence of a paraprotein. An autoantibody screen revealed a weakly positive antinuclear antibody with no specific antibodies against double-stranded DNA or extractable nuclear antigens. Rheumatoid factor was negative. Chest X-ray and electrocardiogram were normal. Urine microscopy and analysis showed an inactive sediment with a trace of proteinuria.

Nerve conduction studies revealed an absent right median sensory nerve action potential (SNAP). The left ulnar and both sural SNAPs were also absent. Other SNAPs were present but reduced (right radial 7 μV, left radial 5 μV, right ulnar 2 μV, left median (index finger) 3 μV). No response was obtained from abductor pollicis brevis stimulating the right median nerve. Though the compound muscle action potentials in the left median motor study were reduced, motor nerve conduction velocity and distal motor latency were normal. Similarly, in the right leg, no response was obtained from extensor digitorum brevis. However, recording from abductor hallucis, tibial motor nerve conduction velocity and distal motor latency were normal. Electromyography showed changes of chronic partial denervation with fibrillation and positive sharp waves in right abductor pollicis brevis and tibialis anterior. A diagnostic procedure was performed.

∗   ∗   ∗

Discussion

This patient's neurological symptoms and signs, and the results of nerve conduction studies, clearly indicate lesions of several peripheral nerves. Thus, the initial right foot-drop is attributable to common peroneal nerve damage. She subsequently developed a right median nerve lesion, involving the anterior interosseous branch, but sparing more proximal injury, as weakness of flexor digitorum superficialis is not mentioned (Fig. 1.2). A mild left ulnar sensory neuropathy then appeared. Finally, she suffered a severe peripheral nerve lesion, presumably sciatic albeit partial, in the left leg.

This asymmetrical pattern, with stepwise deterioration, is characteristic of a multifocal neuropathy, formerly termed mononeuritis multiplex. It is readily distinguishable from the distal symmetrical pattern, with steady progression, of a more typical polyneuropathy. Eventually, however, the multifocal quality may be lost, as peripheral nerve lesions accumulate and become confluent. This was beginning to happen in this case, as evidenced by the sensory loss in the lower limbs on examination, which had assumed a symmetrical stocking distribution.

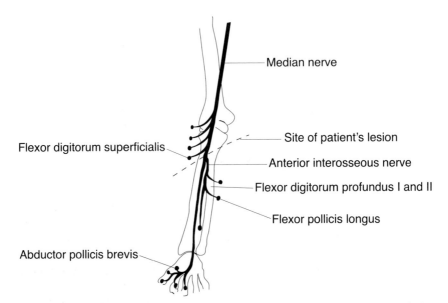

Fig. 1.2. Muscles supplied by the median nerve, showing the site of the patient's lesion.

Table 1.2. Causes of multifocal neuropathy.

Hereditary
  Hereditary neuropathy with liability to pressure palsies.
Infectious
  Leprosy
  Lyme disease
  HIV
Ischemic
  Diabetes
  Vasculitis
  Atherosclerosis
Inflammatory
  Chronic inflammatory demyelinating polyneuropathy
  Multifocal motor neuropathy
  Sarcoidosis
Other
  Carcinoma
  Lymphoma
  Amyloid

The causes of a multifocal neuropathy are summarized in Table 1.2. Of these, many may readily be eliminated immediately. Thus, an inherited disorder (hereditary neuropathy with liability to pressure palsies, HNPP) seems unlikely given the age of onset and subacute progressive presentation. Similarly, infective causes may be excluded in the absence of risk factors and of associated supportive clinical features. Metabolic causes, such as diabetes mellitus, are ruled out by the screening blood tests. The initial investigations also provide no definite evidence for an underlying malignancy, though nonspecific abnormalities, such as the deranged liver function tests, raise this possibility.

The time course of the clinical presentation, progressing over 6 weeks, is perhaps most suggestive of an inflammatory process. More specifically, the stepwise pattern points to a vasculitis, inflammation of the vasa nervorum resulting in repeated ischemic events in the peripheral nerves. Other inflammatory causes are less likely. Thus, there were no specific systemic features of sarcoidosis and the chest X-ray was normal. Multifocal motor neuropathy is a condition which is often confined to the upper limbs. As its name implies, the presence of sensory findings in this patient would argue strongly against such a diagnosis. Furthermore, the electrodiagnostic hallmark of multifocal motor neuropathy, namely conduction block, was not found.

Vasculitic neuropathy may be part of a multi-organ systemic disorder. It may also occur in isolation – tissue-specific or nonsystemic vasculitic neuropathy.[1] The presence of serological markers of inflammation, particularly the grossly abnormal sedimentation rate and C-reactive protein, is

Table 1.3. Systemic disorders associated with vasculitic neuropathy.

Primary vasculitis
  Classical polyarteritis nodosa
  Churg–Strauss syndrome
  Wegener's granulomatosis
  Giant cell arteritis
Autoimmune disease with associated vasculitis
  Rheumatoid arthritis
  Systemic lupus erythematosus
  Sjögren's syndrome
  Cryoglobulinemia
Secondary vasculitis
  – associated with malignancy, serum sickness,
  hypersensitivity or infection

more suggestive of a multisystem disease in this patient. Systemic vasculitides associated with multifocal neuropathy are listed in Table 1.3. Again, many may be excluded by the absence of associated clinical features. Thus, the patient had no evidence of systemic autoimmune disease, e.g. rheumatoid arthritis or systemic lupus erythematosus. Among the primary vasculitides, Churg–Strauss syndrome is precluded by the absence of asthma and eosinophilia. Though the elevated sedimentation rate and C-reactive protein bring giant cell arteritis to mind, similar abnormalities are found in the other systemic vasculitides. The patient's symptoms were not suggestive of giant cell arteritis and multifocal neuropathy is only seen in a small minority of patients with this diagnosis. This leaves Wegeners granulomatosis and classical polyarteritis nodosa as the differential diagnosis. Of these, the former is more probable in the light of the patient's antecedent illnesses, preceding the onset of the neuropathy (see below), and her facial appearance (Fig. 1.1).

Wegeners granulomatosis is a multisystem disease of unknown etiology characterized pathologically by necrotizing vasculitis and granulomatous inflammation. The primary organs affected are the upper and/or lower respiratory tract and the kidneys. Otitis media and hearing loss, as observed in this patient, are typical early features. Involvement of the eyes is also common, including conjunctivitis, iritis, scleritis and granulomatous inflammation of retrobulbar structures. The paranasal sinuses are affected in over 90% of patients. The nasal epithelium and cartilage are also very commonly damaged, with the development of mucosal ulceration and saddle-nose deformity (Fig. 1.1). The patient's renal involvement was presumably mild, given the modest abnormalities on blood and urine testing. Many patients with Wegeners granulomatosis have frank glomerulonephritis or renal vasculitis. Disease of the lower respiratory tract is also often much more severe than that seen in this patient, with pneumonitis, pleurisy, pulmonary hemorrhage and pneumothorax.

Neurological manifestations of Wegeners granulomatosis include cranial nerve palsies and external ophthalmoplegia due to granulomatous infiltration of the orbit or cavernous sinus, aseptic meningitis and intracranial venous sinus thrombosis. Peripheral (multifocal) neuropathy is seen in 10–20% of patients.[2]

Though the etiology of Wegeners granulomatosis remains obscure, there have been advances in understanding its pathogenesis. Most notably, circulating antibodies against neutrophil cytoplasmic components (ANCA) have been demonstrated in this disease.[3] The first diagnostic procedure in the patient under discussion was therefore to assay for these antibodies, which were indeed found to be present in high titer. Antineutrophil cytoplasmic autoantibodies show three staining patterns on cellular assay. First, diffuse cytoplasmic staining (C-ANCA) is seen in >80% of patients with Wegeners granulomatosis and multisystem involvement, though it is also observed in polyarteritis nodosa and focal necrotizing glomerulonephritis. Most C-ANCA antibodies are directed against proteinase 3, a neutral serine proteinase. Perinuclear staining (P-ANCA) is less specific than C-ANCA and may be seen in many autoimmune disorders. The antibodies themselves are directed against a range of neutrophil enzymes, including myeloperoxidase. The third pattern, atypical perinuclear staining, is even less specific and may be seen in both autoimmune and infectious diseases. The potential importance of ANCA as a humoral pathogenetic mechanism for mediating vessel damage in vasculitis is underlined by the fact that ANCA titers correlate with disease activity.[4] However, cell-mediated mechanisms must also be relevant to the pathogenesis of Wegener's granulomatosis, given the presence of granulomas and of a predominance of T lymphocytes and macrophages in lesions.[5]

The second diagnostic procedure was combined peripheral nerve and muscle biopsy, to achieve a histological diagnosis. There is evidence that sampling both nerve and muscle increases the probability of histological proof of systemic vasculitis in patients with multifocal neuropathy, compared to biopsy of only one tissue.[6] In this patient's case, sural nerve fascicular biopsy revealed extensive axonal degeneration (in keeping with the electrodiagnostic findings) but no specific features of vasculitis. However, vasculitic changes and early granuloma formation were detected on the muscle biopsy (Fig. 1.3). Subjecting the patient to these biopsies, in addition to serological investigations, was justified, indeed considered virtually mandatory, on the grounds that she was likely to be embarking on long-term immunosuppressant treatment with potent drugs.

The treatment of Wegeners granulomatosis has been revolutionized by the use of cyclophosphamide, often in combination with corticosteroids.[7] Cyclophosphamide may be administered continuously orally or as pulsed therapy (orally or intravenously). This patient was successfully treated with continuous oral cyclophosphamide (2 mg/kg daily) for 12 months in

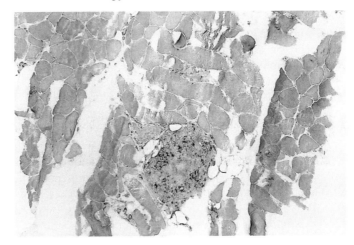

Fig. 1.3. Muscle biopsy, stained for acid phosphatase, showing macrophage infiltration around blood vessels (×100).

combination with corticosteroids (initially methylprednisolone 1 g intrave-nously daily for 3 days then reducing doses of oral prednisolone). After 12 months, immunosuppression was maintained with azathioprine (2 mg/kg daily) and low-dose prednisolone. She became ambulant again, with the use of two sticks, and the upper limb mononeuropathies resolved.

Diagnosis

Multifocal neuropathy secondary to Wegeners granulomatosis.

References

1. Dyck PJ, Benstead TJ, Conn DL et al. Nonsystemic vasculitic neuropathy. *Brain* 1987; **110**: 843–853.
2. Nishino H, Rubino FA, DeRemee RA et al. Neurological involvement in Wegener's granulomatosis: an analysis of 324 consecutive patients at the Mayo Clinic. *Ann Neurol* 1993; **33**: 4–9.
3. Goeken JA. Antineutrophil cytoplasmic antibody – a useful serological marker for vasculitis. *J Clin Immunol* 1991; **11**: 161–174.
4. Egner W, Chapel HM. Titration of antibodies against neutrophil cytoplasmic antigens is useful in monitoring disease activity in systemic vasculitides. *Clin Exp Immunol* 1990; **82**: 244–249.
5. Gephardt GN, Ahmad M, Tubbs RR. Pulmonary vasculitis (Wegener's granu-lomatosis). Immunohistochemical study of T and B cell markers. *Am J Med* 1983; **74**: 700–704.
6. Said G, Lacroix-Ciaudo C, Fujimura H et al. The peripheral neuropathy of necrotizing arteritis: a clinicopathological study. *Ann Neurol* 1988; **23**: 461–465.
7. Fauci AS, Katz P, Haynes BF, Wolff SM Cyclophosphamide therapy of severe systemic necrotizing vasculitis. *N Engl J Med* 1979; **301**: 235–238.

Rapid onset of depression, mutism and rigidity

Clinical history and examination

JZ is a 33-year-old, married woman. She was admitted to a psychiatric unit of a tertiary care hospital with a diagnosis of depression. Before she became ill, she had been caring for a grandmother with Alzheimers disease and a 12-year-old son; she managed all aspects of her home. Six weeks prior to admission, her grandmother died. The patient acted in a strange and uncharacteristic manner at the funeral. She seemed inappropriate, and her behavior became increasingly unusual thereafter. She became withdrawn, taciturn, and answered questions in an odd fashion. Two days prior to admission, she stopped eating and seemed confused. She needed help to eat and dress, and was incontinent of urine.

On admission she was alert but mute. She answered questions by nodding her head, but the responses came very slowly. Most responses were appropriate. During the first 4–5 days on the psychiatric unit, her behavior deteriorated, and computed tomography (CT) revealed multiple ring-enhancing lesions in the white matter of both cerebral hemispheres, extending to the junction with the corpus callosum. The cerebellum and brainstem were unaffected.

She was transferred to the medical service, where she was mute and rigid. Tendon reflexes were exaggerated and extensor plantar responses and bilateral grasp reflexes were present. Cranial MRI (Fig. 2.1) showed multiple, large, rounded and confluent areas of abnormal increased signal intensity in the white matter of both cerebral hemispheres, involving all lobes including the lateral margins of the temporal white matter. Posterior fossa and brainstem structures were spared. A small area of increased signal was seen in the region of the genu of the right internal capsule. There was little mass effect, and ventricular size was normal. There was no enhancement following gadolinium DTPA administration.

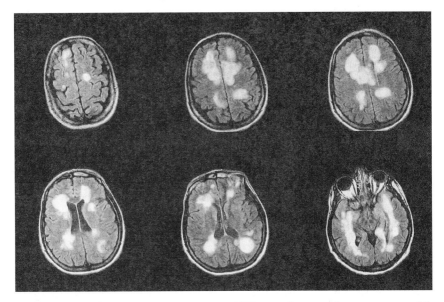

Fig. 2.1. Axial FLAIR images from brain MRI scan. Images demonstrate multiple large round lesions in the periventricular and axial white matter. There was no enhancement following gadolinium administration (not shown).

Total protein, albumin, calcium, bilirubin, alkaline phosphatase, ALT, AST, glucose, BUN, creatinine, electrolytes and CBC were normal. B12 level was 280 pg/ml, WSR was 19, CRP 0.4, PT and PTT normal, free T_4 1.1, TSH 1.84, ANA positive at a titer of 1:320, anti-single stranded DNA normal (25), anti-Sm antibody negative, Toxoplasma IgG and IgM antibody negative, RPR negative, HTLV-1 antibody negative, Lyme IgG/IgM antibody normal (0.31), HIV-1 antibody EIA non-reactive, and multiple blood cultures were negative.

The cerebrospinal fluid had 14 cells/μl, 75% of which were lymphocytes. Cerebrospinal fluid protein was 80 mg %, glucose was 81 mg %, IgG index was 0.71 (normal 0.67), IgG synthesis rate was increased (16.2 mg/24 h), and oligoclonal bands were present. A stereotactic biopsy was taken from the right frontal lobe on the 10th hospital day, about 7 weeks after the onset of behavioral changes.

Pathology

Stereotactic biopsies from the right frontal lobe region were examined histologically. Biopsies consisted of white matter tissue. Demyelination was evident on a luxol fast blue stain. Areas of demyelination were marked by prominent macrophage infiltrates, associated with gliosis and perivascular lymphocytic infiltrates (Figs 2.2 and 2.3). A Bodian stain showed relative preservation of axons in areas of myelin loss. Alzheimer type I astrocytes and viral inclusions were not identified. There was no

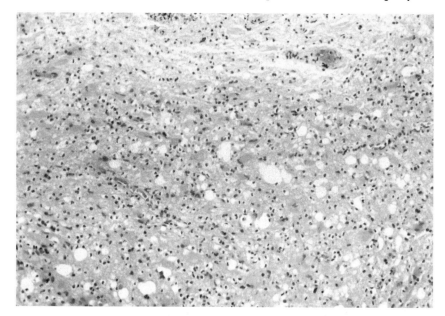

Fig. 2.2. White matter marked by infiltrating macrophages and reactive astrocytes. (Hematoxylin and eosin, original magnification ×200.)

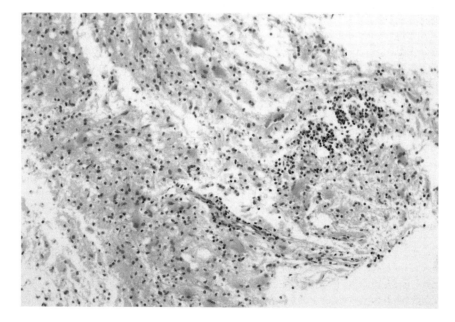

Fig. 2.3. Prominent perivascular lymphocytic infiltrate associated with a demyelinating lesion. (Hematoxylin and eosin, original magnification ×200.)

evidence of neoplasia. The histopathologic findings were consistent with those seen with active inflammatory demyelination.

Treatment and course

Following the brain biopsy, the patient was treated with intravenous methylprednisolone, 1000 mg daily for 3 days, without improvement. She remained awake but mute, unable to follow commands, unable to feed herself or walk, and incontinent. She had exaggerated tendon reflexes, upgoing toes, and grasp reflexes. Starting on the 14th hospital day, she was given a 5-day course of intravenous cyclophosphamide, 750 mg per day, and intravenous methylprednisolone, 1000 mg per day.

She tolerated cyclophosphamide therapy well, and was discharged on the 20th hospital day to a nursing home, where her condition gradually improved, and she was discharged to home 3 months after the first admission. Two months later, she was living with her husband and 13-year-old son. Her husband and son provided needed supervision along with her parents. She was ambulatory and could care for herself to some extent. She had difficulty controlling her bladder, but was continent. Mood swings ranged from angry and loud to happily manic. On examination, she was hyperkinetic, moving about the room constantly. She attended to the examiner, and followed directions. She tended to hug and kiss people in the room with great fanfare. Speech was effusive with frequent perseverations. Much of the speech had no purpose. She could not accurately state the year, name the month, or name any month, until her mother asked her 'What comes after January?' She then rattled off the months, but finally settled incorrectly on December as the current month. She did not know the day, place, or situation. To the question, 'What is your medical condition?' she replied, 'You are the king.' When informed of her diagnosis, she said 'OK, OK, OK, everyone knows that' and then continued on with a different subject. She tended to confabulate throughout the interview. She could name objects, and volunteered their functions extensively. She could not add or subtract. She could identify her right hand, but not the examiner's right hand. She had no long tract signs. She was started on interferon beta therapy.

Her exam 7 months later (approximately 1 year after the onset symptoms) showed continuing improvement. Her behavior was more appropriate, and she was fully oriented. Her husband indicated that she required much less supervision, and spent much of her time alone at home.

*   *   *

Discussion

The differential diagnosis at the time of initial evaluation included lymphoma, progressive multifocal leukoencephalopathy, infection, or demyelinating conditions such as acute disseminated encephalomyelitis or acute progressive multiple sclerosis. On brain biopsy, there were no atypical lymphoid cells, as would be seen with lymphoma, or Cowdry A viral inclusions within oligodendrocytes, as in progressive multifocal leukoencephalopathy.

The histopathologic findings of white matter myelin loss accompanied by macrophages, reactive astrocytosis and a benign perivascular lymphoid infiltrate supported a diagnosis of inflammatory demyelination, such as acute disseminated encephalomyelitis (ADEM) or acute progressive multiple sclerosis. Distinction on routine light microscopic grounds between these two entities may be difficult. Typically, ADEM preferentially involves perivascular white matter and becomes confluent with time. In the hyperacute stage, petecheal hemorrhages and thrombosis of small white matter vessels may be seen.

The clinical course, MRI findings, and CSF findings were more consistent with acute progressive MS than with ADEM. ADEM and its hyperacute form, acute necrotizing hemorrhagic encephalopathy (ANHE), are thought to be forms of immunemediated inflammatory demyelination. These disorders are typically monophasic, while MS is, by definition, multiphasic or chronically progressive. Patients with ADEM or ANHE usually have fever, headache, meningeal signs and altered consciousness, manifestations that are exceedingly rare in patients with MS.

In ADEM, there is commonly an antecedent event, most commonly a viral illness or inoculation, followed days or weeks later by an acute monophasic disseminated disease of the CNS. Pathologically, there are features of perivascular inflammation and demyelination. The most commonly recognized antecedent event is a viral infection or inoculation. ADEM is more frequent after exposure to certain viruses, particularly RNA viruses that bud from infected cells. Antecedent infections include measles,[1,2] rubella,[3] varicella,[4] mumps,[5] influenza,[6] Herpes simplex,[7] or viruses causing nonspecific upper respiratory infections. Measles is the viral infection most commonly complicated by ADEM.[2] On occasion the syndrome follows vaccination for rubella, pertussis, influenza, or vaccinia, and it commonly follows rabies inoculation.[8] Drugs have been related to the syndrome.[9,10] This patient had no evident precipitating event, although that does not rule out ADEM.

Clinical features in this case were distinctly unusual for ADEM. Typically, nonspecific symptoms of fever, headache, anorexia, and vomiting are rapidly followed by meningeal signs, altered consciousness, and focal signs referable to brain, spinal cord, optic nerves, or spinal roots. Neurological signs are often multiplex, consisting of some combination of pyramidal tract dysfunction, cranial nerve signs, movement disorders, sensory system dysfunction, cerebellar signs, seizures, and loss of muscle stretch responses. Certain clinical features are more commonly associated with specific antecedent events. For example, an acute cerebellar syndrome commonly follows varicella zoster infection; myoclonus commonly accompanies ADEM after measles infection; and hemiplegia is particularly common following mumps infection.

The CSF in ADEM may be under increased pressure, and usually contains a slight mononuclear cell pleocytosis and moderate protein elevation, although CSF is normal in 20–30% of cases. There may be normal[11] or increased[12] IgG levels.

The principal condition to be distinguished from ADEM in this case is MS. The patient clearly does not have typical relapsing remitting MS. Acute progressive MS (Marburg disease)[13] refers to a patient with no prior history of MS who develops acute or subacute progressive neurologic deterioration and severe disability within days to months. As initially described, patients progress steadily to a quadriplegic obtunded state with death due to intercurrent infection, aspiration or respiratory failure. Post-mortem studies have documented inflammation in the optic nerves, optic chiasm, cerebral hemispheres, and spinal cord.

This patient seems to have had acute progressive MS, but the explanation for her recovery is not certain. Kurtzke[14] reported on the characteristics of 220 MS patients following an acute relapse. The patients were primarily men in military service who were observed in a hospital. None of them were treated with corticosteroids or ACTH. Only 14% of patients with a relapse that progressed for over 1 month subsequently improved. This pattern suggests that our patient improved as a result of treatment with methylprednisolone and cyclophosphamide, rather than by natural history. She was treated with interferon beta to prevent recurrent relapses, but the risk of future relapses could not be estimated with confidence.

Diagnosis

Multiple sclerosis.

References

1. Boughton CR. Morbilli in Sydney: Part II. Neurological sequelae of morbilli. *Med J Aust* 1964; **2**: 908–915.
2. Johnson R, Griffin D, Hirsch J et al. Measles encephalomyelitis: clinical and immunological studies. *N Engl J Med* 1984; **310**: 137–141.
3. Sherman FE, Michaels RH, Kenny FM. Acute encephalopathy (encephalitis) complicating rubella. *JAMA* 1965; **192**: 675–681.
4. Miller HG, Stanton JB, Gibbons JL. Parainfectious encephalomyelitis and related syndromes. A critical review of neurologic complications of certain specific fevers. *Q J Med* 1956; **25**: 427–505.
5. Donohue WL, Playfair FD, Whitaker L. Mumps encephalitis, pathology and pathogenesis. *J Pediatr* 1955; **47**: 395–412.
6. Flewett TH, Hoult JG. Influenzal encephalopathy and post influenzal encephalitis. *Lancet* 1958; **2**: 11–15.

7. Koenig H, Rabinowitz SG, Day E, Miller V. Post-infectious encephalomyelitis after successful treatment of herpes simplex encephalitis with adenine arabino-side. *N Engl J Med* 1979; **300**: 1089–1093.
8. Scott TFM. Postinfectious and vaccinal encephalitis. *Med Clin North Am* 1967; **51**: 701–717.
9. Adams RD, Cammermeyer J, Denny-Brown D. Acute necrotizing hemorrhagic encephalopathy. *J Neuropathol Exp Neurol* 1949; **8**: 1–28.
10. Cavanagh JB. Encephalopathy following administration of streptomycin and para-aminosalicyclic acid. *J Clin Pathol* 1953; **6**: 128–131.
11. Johnson KP, Wolinsky JS, Ginsberg AH. Immune mediated syndromes of the nervous system related to virus infection. In: Vinken PJ, Bruyn GW, Klawans HL, eds. *Handbook of Clinical Neurology*. New York: Elsevier, 1978: 391–434.
12. Skoldenberg B, Carlstrom A, Forsgren M, Norrby E. Transient appearance of oligoclonal immunoglobulin and measles virus antibodies in the cerebrospinal fluid in a case of acute measles encephalitis. *Clin Exp Immunol* 1976; **23**: 451–455.
13. Johnson MD, Lavin P, Whetsell WO. Fulminant monophasic multiple sclerosis, Marburg's type. *J Neurol Neurosurg Psych* 1990; **53**: 918–921.
14. Kurtzke JF. Course of exacerbations of multiple sclerosis in hospitalized patients. *Arch Neurol* 2000; **76**: 175–184.

Sudden onset hemiparesis

Clinical history and examination

A 46-year-old woman was admitted to the hospital because of sudden left hemiparesis. Except for a history of asthma, uterine fibroid, and 'headaches for years,' she was well until 4 hours prior to admission, when she suddenly developed a severe right temporal headache ('the worst headache of my life') and difficulty moving her left side. Paramedics found her blood pressure to be 190/110 mmHg and her pulse 100 and regular. She was 'alert and oriented ×3,' with left facial droop, left hemiparesis, and slurred speech. The Emergency Medical Service brought her to the hospital.

There was no prior history of hypertension, diabetes mellitus, or cardiac disease. She took oral contraceptive pills as treatment for menorrhagia secondary to uterine fibroids, diagnosed 2 months earlier. Asthma, treated intermittently with an albuterol sulfate nebulizer, had begun 20 years before, following a bout of pneumonia. Intermittent headaches for many years were mild and did not resemble her current headache. She had smoked a pack of cigarettes daily for 30 years. She denied alcohol abuse or illicit drug use.

In the emergency room her blood pressure was 160/102 mmHg, pulse 93 per minute and regular, respiratory rate 20 per minute and regular, and temperature 97F. Findings on general physical examination were normal except for mild diffuse pulmonary rhonchi. Her neck was not stiff. She was alert and mildly inattentive, complaining of headache and nausea, but she cooperated with the examination and could count backward from 20 to 1. There was left hemineglect; she ignored instructions delivered from her left side, she bisected a line markedly to the right of midline, and she omitted the left half of copied diagrams. She did not acknowledge her left hemiparesis, and she identified her left arm as belonging to the examiner. Orientation and memory were intact, as was verbal expression, speech comprehension, naming, repetition, oral reading, calculation, and praxis.

Left homonymous hemianopia was probably present. Fundi were normal, and pupils were equal and reactive. There was mild right ptosis. Her eye movements were conjugate, but she did not bring her eyes past midline to the left, either spontaneously or when pursuing a target; with the oculocephalic maneuver the eyes moved conjugately past the midline to the left. Left facial weakness spared the forehead, and she was dysarthric, with deviation of her tongue to the left. Her left arm and leg had 3/5 strength proximally and 0/5 strength distally. Muscle tone was not increased, but tendon reflexes were slightly brisker in the left limbs, and the left plantar response was extensor. Gross touch and pinprick sensation were recognized throughout but decreased on the left.

Hematocrit was 24%, hemoglobin 7.3 g/dl, mean corpuscular volume (MCV) 69 fl, mean corpuscular hemoglobin (MCH) 21 pg/cell, and mean corpuscular hemoglobin concentration 30.4 g/dl. White blood count was 6100/mm^3 (50% polymorphonuclears, 35% lymphocytes, 8% monocytes, 7% eosinophils). Platelets were 509 000/mm^3. Reticulocytes were 0.6%. Serum ferritin was 4.1 ng/ml. Urinalysis was normal except for the presence of many red blood cells. Blood glucose was 136 mg/dl. Serum sodium, potassium, chloride, bicarbonate, urea nitrogen, creatinine, total protein, albumin, calcium, phosphorus, magnesium, cholesterol, uric acid, bilirubin, alkaline phosphatase, lactate dehydrogenase, cobalamin, thyroid-stimulating hormone, and creatine kinase were normal. Urine was positive for cocaine metabolites and negative for amphetamines, barbiturates, opiates, methadone, benzodiazepines, cannabinoids, and phencyclidine. Hepatitis B core and surface antibodies and surface antigen were negative. Arterial pO$_2$ was 74 mmHg and O$_2$ saturation 95.3%; arterial pH was 7.45, pCO$_2$ 34.5 mmHg, and bicarbonate 23.8 mmol/l. Prothrombin time and partial thromboplastin time were normal.

Electrocardiography revealed NEA and flattening of T waves in leads I, II, aVF, V5, and V6. Chest radiograph was normal. Serum troponin was normal. Transthoracic echocardiography showed moderate concentric left ventricular hypertrophy with normal global systolic function; no thrombus was seen.

Computed tomography (CT) of the head without contrast showed patchy areas of early infarction in the territory of distal right middle cerebral artery branches (Fig. 3.1). Cerebrospinal fluid (CSF) was clear and colorless with normal pressure, no white blood cells, 50 red blood cells/mm^3, protein 22 mg/dl, and glucose 88 mg/dl.

During her second hospital day she was mildly lethargic and still complained of headache, which now spread to her right retro-orbital area and neck. Her left limbs were flaccid and paralyzed. She still had left hemineglect but now recognized her left limbs as her own. Anhidrosis was present over her right face, her right pupil was slightly smaller than her left, and there continued to be mild right-sided ptosis. Repeat CT of the head showed more obvious evidence of infarction in the territory of the

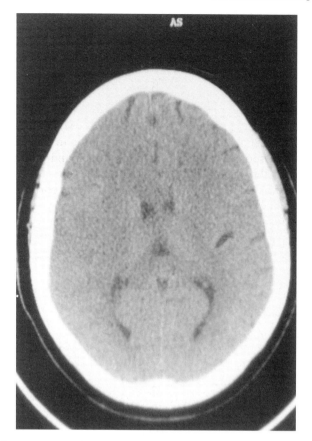

Fig. 3.1. Computed tomography scan showing right cerebral swelling, with subtle lucency and sulcal obliteration, suggestive of infarction. (Courtesy Dr Paoula Bowers.)

right middle and anterior cerebral arteries; there was no hemorrhagic transformation (Fig. 3.2).

A diagnostic study was performed.

*   *   *

Discussion

This woman's clinical presentation – a sudden severe headache unlike any she had previously experienced, with left hemiparesis and hemineglect – makes spontaneous intracranial hemorrhage, particularly subarachnoid hemorrhage secondary to a ruptured saccular aneurysm, the working

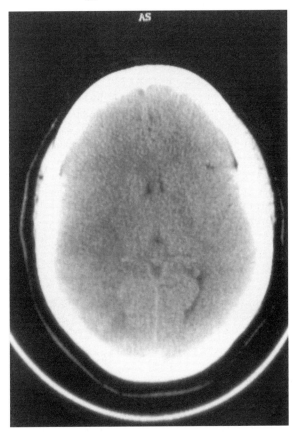

Fig. 3.2. Repeat CT, 1 day after the first, showing more obvious and extensive cerebral swelling, with right-to-left shift of the lateral ventricles and lucency in the territory of the right middle and anterior cerebral arteries. (Courtesy Dr Paoula Bowers.)

diagnosis until proven otherwise. She had several risk factors for such an event. She smoked tobacco, and she had recently begun taking oral contraceptive drugs (for menorrhagia secondary to uterine fibroid). Although she reported normal blood pressure, it was elevated on admission, perhaps an artifact of acute discomfort and anxiety or perhaps reflecting a hypertensive state undetected in the past. Her admission platelet count was mildly elevated.

She denied illicit drug use, yet her urine contained cocaine metabolites. Such metabolites tend to persist for a few days after a single dose of cocaine; in heavy daily users (in particular smokers of alkaloidal 'crack' cocaine) urine metabolites can persist for a few weeks. Both intracerebral and subarachnoid hemorrhage are recognized complications of cocaine use, and in such patients saccular aneurysms and vascular malformations are often found at cerebral angiography.[1] Intracranial hemorrhage temporally associated with cocaine use is probably the result of a hypertensive surge associated with the drug.

On admission she had left hemiparesis and facial weakness, which indicated a lesion of the corticospinal/corticobulbar system above the level of the seventh nerve nucleus in the pons, and left hemineglect, anosognosia, and asomatognosia, which indicated a lesion of the right cerebral hemisphere, most likely the parietal lobe. Her severe hemineglect made interpretation of visual field and sensory testing difficult, but she seemed to have left homonymous hemianopia, reflecting damage to the visual pathway behind the optic chiasm on the right (optic tract, lateral geniculate nucleus of the thalamus, optic radiations, or visual cortex in the occipital lobe). A ruptured saccular aneurysm arising from branching of the middle cerebral artery within the sylvian fissure could acutely produce this constellation of signs secondary to hematoma formation. It could produce similar signs as a result of vasospasm and ischemia, but vasospasm secondary to subarachnoid hemorrhage does not usually appear until 2 or 3 (or more) days later.

CT revealed early evidence of infarction in the territory of right middle cerebral artery distal branches but no blood either intraparenchymally or in subarachnoid spaces. Absence of intracranial blood at CT does not exclude subarachnoid hemorrhage, and so a spinal tap was performed. Only 50 red blood cells/mm^3 were present, the fluid was clear and colorless, and the protein content was normal; a mild elevation of glucose content reflected a mildly elevated blood glucose level.

Diagnostic considerations thus shifted from possible spontaneous intracranial hemorrhage to right middle cerebral artery territory infarction with an unusually severe right-sided headache. Cocaine use could still have been contributory. Cocaine causes ischemic stroke (and myocardial infarction) probably by direct vasoconstriction.[2] Cocaine can also cause cardiac arrhythmia or cardiomyopathy with secondary cardioembolism.[3] Cardiac workup, including electrocardiogram, serum troponin level, and transthoracic echocardiography failed to identity an embolic source, however.

Headache is a frequent accompaniment of cerebral infarction, both thrombotic and embolic. The patient had had previous headaches, not characterized in detail but different, at least in severity, from her present headache. Stroke is an infrequent complication of migraine, and the mechanism is uncertain.[4] Primary vasospasm is no longer considered the cause of migrainous aura; rather, vasoconstriction appears to be secondary to underlying cerebral hypometabolism. One possibility is that ischemic stroke occurs when such vasoconstriction, even though an autoregulatory response, is sufficient to cause sludging, platelet aggregation, and thrombosis. (By contrast, the hemiplegia of familial hemiplegic migraine is the result of a central nervous system channelopathy involving calcium channels.[5])

On the patient's second hospital day pain was present in her right head and neck and a right-sided Horner syndrome became more obvious. The most ready explanation for unilateral head and neck pain, Horner syndrome, and cerebral infarction would be carotid artery dissection.

Over two-thirds of patients with ischemic stroke secondary to cervico-cerebral arterial dissection are between 35 and 50 years of age.[6] The usual symptoms are those of stroke or transient ischemic attack associated with ipsilateral head, face, or neck pain, which can precede the ischemic symptoms by hours or days.[7] Some patients experience a subjective bruit, and some develop neuropathies of lower cranial nerves, especially the hypoglossal, as a result of expansion of subadventitial dissection within the cervical parapharyngeal space.[8] In some cases pain and Horner syndrome exist without ischemic symptoms.[9]

Traumatic precipitation includes chiropractic manipulation and anesthesia administration with hyperextension of the neck, but trauma may be minimal (e.g. nose-blowing) or absent.[6] Fibromuscular dysplasia is present in about 15% of cases and hypertension in about a quarter. Other associated conditions include Marfan syndrome, Ehlers–Danlos syndrome, systemic lupus erythematosus, atherosclerotic plaques, and migraine. Cystic medial necrosis is often present histologically.[10–12]

Luminal stenosis follows subintimal hemorrhage, whereas arterial dilatation follows subadventitial hemorrhage. In some cases a primary intimal tear is probably the initial event, and in others intimal tear follows primary intramedial hemorrhage. Ischemic symptoms are most often secondary to distal embolism of local thrombi rather than to lumenal narrowing.[12–14]

Cervical carotid dissection usually begins 2 cm or more distal to the origin of the internal carotid artery and terminates before the artery's entry into the petrous bone. Dissection in the common carotid artery or the intracranial carotid and middle cerebral arteries is much less frequent. Extracranial carotid sonography, which most reliably images the carotid bifurcation, can miss lesions above and below. More sensitive is angiography, which most often shows irregular narrowing of the artery; sometimes there is a tapered occlusion or an 'extraluminal pouch.'[13] Magnetic resonance imaging (MRI) and magnetic resonance angiography (MRA) have the advantage over conventional angiography of showing the vessel in cross-section, which can reveal a double lumen ('crescent sign'). In one report of carotid dissection, MRA had a sensitivity of 95% and a specificity of 99%, and other reports describe detection by MRI of carotid dissections missed by conventional angiography.[15,16]

Extracranial carotid dissection causes moderate-to-severe neurological impairment in less than a third of cases.[13] Extension of extracranial dissection intracranially is rare. Primary intracranial carotid dissection produces major neurological impairment or death in the majority of cases, and in 20%, rupture through the adventitia causes subarachnoid hemorrhage.[17]

Dissection also affects the vertebral artery, often with cervical or occipital pain and stroke, especially lateral medullary or cerebellar infarction.[18] As with carotid artery dissection, intracranial extension of vertebral artery dissection carries a high risk for subarachnoid hemorrhage.[19] Primary dissection of the basilar artery is rare.[13]

Although randomized clinical trials are lacking, the likely mechanism of ischemic stroke in most extracranial cervicocerebral dissections – i.e. local thrombosis and distal embolism – favors acute treatment with heparin or a heparinoid agent.[13] Alternatively, antiplatelet drugs or, if less than a few hours have elapsed since onset of symptoms, intra-arterial administration of a thrombolytic agent might be considered. The appearance of the lesion on subsequent MRI and MRA imaging would then influence the decision to continue anticoagulation therapy or to switch to an antiplatelet agent. Surgical approaches include aneurysm resection and arterial reconstruction.

This patient's clinical picture was entirely consistent with carotid artery dissection. Moreover, the loss of sweating over the right side of her face favored dissection of the common carotid rather than the internal carotid artery, for sympathetic fibers mediating facial sweating travel into the face along the external carotid artery, in contrast to sympathetic fibers headed for the orbit, which travel along the internal carotid artery. An appropriate study at this point would be MRI and MRA.

Further discussion

MRI and MRA were incomplete because the patient developed claustrophobia and the procedure had to be terminated. MRA axial cuts, however, revealed a probable double lumen of the right common carotid artery, consistent with dissection (Fig. 3.3).

Doppler ultrasound examination of the neck at the level of the common carotid artery bifurcation and proximal internal carotid artery did not show the dissection.

The patient received heparin in dosage to maintain partial thromboplastin time (PTT) below 45 seconds. There was no gross vaginal bleeding, but occasional increases in her microscopic hematuria led to temporary reduction of heparin dosage. Over the next several days the asomatognosia cleared, but left hemiplegia and facial weakness persisted, and there continued to be evidence of left hemineglect, with failure to acknowledge her left-sided paralysis. Oral anticoagulation with warfarin was then added, aiming for a prothrombin time INR of 2 to 3. Eleven days after admission, heparin was discontinued. Iron replacement therapy was given for her iron deficiency anemia. Attempts to obtain a better image of the right carotid artery were unsuccessful.

Diagnosis

Cerebral infarction probably secondary to common carotid artery dissection.

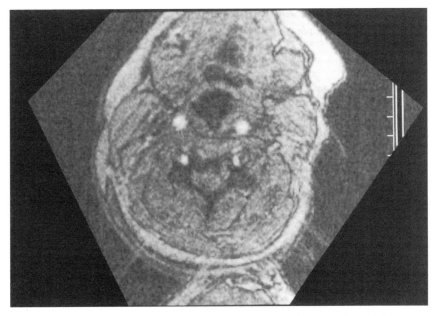

Fig. 3.3. Magnetic resonance angiography image showing, in axial cuts, a probable double lumen of the right common carotid artery, compatible with dissection. (Courtesy Dr Paoula Bowers.)

References

1. Brust JCM. *Neurological Aspects of Substance Abuse.* Boston: Butterworth-Heinemann, 1993.
2. Brust JCM. Stroke and substance abuse. In: Barnett HJM, Mohr JP, Stein BM, Yatsu FM, eds. *Stroke: Pathophysiology, Diagnosis, and Management*, 3rd edn. New York: Churchill-Livingstone, 1998: 979–1000.
3. Petty GW, Brust JCM, Tatemichi TK, Barr ML. Embolic stroke after smoking 'crack' cocaine. *Stroke* 1990; **21**: 1632–1635.
4. Bogousslavsky J, Regli F, Van Melle G et al. Migraine stroke. *Neurology* 1988; **38**: 223–227.
5. Hans M, Luvisetto S, Williams ME et al. Functional consequences of mutations in the human a1A calcium channel subunit linked to familial hemiplegic migraine. *J Neurosci* 1999; **19**: 1610–1619.
6. Hart RG, Easton JD. Dissections of cervical and cerebral arteries. *Neurol Clin* 1983; **1**: 155–182.
7. Biousse V, D'Anglejean-Chatillon J, Massiou H, Bousser M-G. Time course of symptoms in extracranial carotid artery dissections. *Stroke* 1995; **26**: 235–239.
8. Sturzenegger M, Huber P. Cranial nerve palsies in spontaneous carotid artery dissection. *J Neurol Neurosurg Psychiatry* 1993; **56**: 1191–1199.
9. Biousse V, D'Anglejean-Chatillon J, Massiou H, Bousser M-G. Head pain in non-traumatic carotid artery dissection: a series of 65 patients. *Cephalgia* 1994; **14**: 33–36.

10. Sturzenegger M, Mattle HP, Rivoir A, Baumgartner RW. Ultrasound findings in carotid artery dissection: analysis of 43 patients. *Neurology* 1995; **45**: 691–698.
11. Mokri B, Sundt TM, Houser OW, Piepgras DG. Spontaneous dissection of the internal carotid artery. *Ann Neurol* 1986; **19**: 126–138.
12. O'Connell BK, Towfighi J, Brennan RW et al. Dissecting aneurysms of the head and neck. *Neurology* 1985; **35**: 993–997.
13. Saver JL, Easton JD. Dissections and trauma of cervicocerebral arteries. In Barnett HJM, Mohr JP, Stein BM, Yatsu FM, eds. *Stroke: Pathophysiology, Diagnosis, and Management*, 3rd edn. New York: Churchill-Livingstone, 1998: 769–786.
14. Bogousslavsky J, Despland PA, Regli F. Spontaneous carotid dissection with acute stroke. *Arch Neurol* 1987; **44**: 137–140.
15. Levy C, Laissy JP, Reveau V et al. Carotid and vertebral dissections: three-dimensional time of flight MR angiography and MR imaging versus conventional angiography. *Radiology* 1994; **190**: 97–103.
16. Ozdoba C, Sturzenegger M, Schroth G. Internal carotid artery dissection: MR imaging features and clinical radiologic correlation. *Radiology* 1996; **199**: 191–198.
17. Bassetti C, Bogousslavsky J, Eskenasy-Cottier AC et al. Spontaneous intracranial dissection in the anterior circulation. *Cerebrovasc Dis* 1994; **4**: 170–174.
18. Hinse P, Thie A, Lachenmayer L. Dissection of the extracranial vertebral artery: report of four cases and review of the literature. *J Neurol Neurosurg Psychiatry* 1991; **54**: 863–869.
19. Caplan LR, Baquis GD, Pessin MS et al. Dissection of the intracranial vertebral artery. *Neurology* 1988; **38**: 868–877.

Hereditary migraine

Clinical history and examination

A 35-year-old man had a history of stereotyped headaches that began in his early teens. They occurred, on average, every 3 months. The throbbing pain was located in the right or left temple, would peak to maximum intensity within 30 minutes, and was associated with nausea, occasional vomiting, worsening with movement, photophobia, and blurred vision. He had no associated vertigo, ataxia, dysphagia, or tinnitus. The typical headache duration was 10–24 hours. Half of the headaches were associated with right-sided face, arm, and leg weakness that started within 1 hour of headache onset and progressed over 10–20 minutes. The weakness usually lasted 40–60 minutes but could remain throughout the entire duration of the headache and sometimes outlasted the headache by several days. His motor function always returned to normal. With several episodes he developed aphasia, with normal comprehension but paucity of speech. He also had auras of scintillating scotomas that lasted 20–30 minutes, without motor or language dysfunction. Mild head trauma (accidentally hitting his head) could bring on an episode of hemiparesis and headache. Numerous computed tomographic scans, three brain magnetic resonance imagings (MRIs) (two during attacks and one interictally), and one magnetic resonance angiogram of the intracranial and extracranial circulation were normal. He had no other significant medical history, specifically no history of hypertension, hyperlipidemia, arrhythmias, or illegal drug use.

His family history was significant for migraine with prolonged auras in his mother and maternal grandmother. His mother had multiple attacks of hemiparesis followed by typical migraine headaches. Her weakness could last days to weeks, but she never had any permanent residual symptoms. She had not had any episodes of aphasia, but she did have frequent visual auras. Her limited workup included a brain MRI scan and several coagulopathy studies, all of which were within normal limits. She developed an ataxic gait that slowly worsened. The patient's deceased maternal grand-mother had multiple episodes of auras with hemiparesis and aphasia associated with throbbing, severe hemicranial headaches. The family was not aware of any investigative studies she may have had. There was no family history of clotting disorders or multiple miscarriages (suggestive of anti-phospholipid antibody syndrome).

When examined, the patient was symptom-free. His general and neuro-logic examinations were completely normal. Specifically, neurovascular evaluation demonstrated no cardiac murmurs or carotid, cranial, or orbital bruits. He was seen in the emergency department during an attack, and he had a right hemiparesis with face, arm, and leg weakness, and language dysfunction suggesting a Broca's type aphasia. A differential diagnosis was made and investigations organized.

*   *   *

Discussion

The patient had a longstanding history of headaches that fit the International Headache Society (IHS) criteria for migraine with aura and migraine without aura. He had more than five attacks of moderate to severe throbbing pain that worsened with movement and were associated with nausea, vomiting, photophobia, and phonophobia. The patient also experienced auras, which are symptoms of cortical or brainstem dysfunction. These typically lasted from 5 to 60 minutes and were followed by a migraine headache within one hour. He experienced motor, visual, and language auras. The auras could last longer than 60 minutes; thus a better term for them would be prolonged auras. By IHS definition, a prolonged aura lasts for more than 60 minutes but less than 7 days. The patient had two relatives who were known to have migraine associated with prolonged auras and spells of hemiparesis. The family history suggested a maternal inheritance pattern, but, as he was an only child, this may be autosomal inheritance. In addition to episodes of migraine with prolonged aura, his mother had progressive cerebellar dysfunction.

Patients who present with a headache and focal neurologic deficits must be evaluated for transient ischemic attacks and stroke before attributing all of their symptoms to migraine. A diagnosis of repeated transient ischemic attacks is unlikely in our patient because of his young age, the lack of stroke risk factors, the nonacute onset of symptoms, and normal neuro-imaging. The patient's family history of migraine with prolonged aura suggests a familial and genetic cause of his attacks. The apparent maternal inheritance suggests a mitochondrial disorder, such as mitochon-drial encephalomyopathy with lactic acidosis and stroke-like episodes (MELAS), which can present as stroke and migraine in young people.

The patient and his family need to be evaluated for mitochondrial deoxyribonucleic acid (mtDNA) mutations. Another genetic disorder that can present with migraine and stroke is cerebral autosomal dominant arteriopathy with subcortical infarcts and leukoencephalopathy (CADASIL), a non-atherosclerotic, non-amyloid arteriopathy. All symptomatic patients with CADASIL have abnormal neuroimaging (see below). Since our patient had normal MRIs, this diagnosis is excluded. The patient most likely has autosomal dominant familial hemiplegic migraine (FHM), a genetically heterogeneous form of migraine with aura that presents with headache and variable weakness. FHM is a diagnosis of exclusion, i.e. it is diagnosed only after ruling out secondary causes of migraine with prolonged aura.

Patients with prolonged auras should be evaluated for coagulopathies. Lupus anticoagulant, anticardiolipin antibodies, deficiencies in protein C and S, antithrombin III, elevated homocysteine, and the factor V leiden mutation were all negative or normal in our patient. Transesophageal echocardiogram revealed no patent foramen ovale, cardiac valve vegetations, or aortic cholesterol plaques. No mtDNA point mutations or large-scale deletions at the MELAS and myoclonic epilepsy with ragged red fibers (MERRF) genetic loci were found.

Genetics of migraine

Most migraineurs have a strong family history of migraine. Migraine is a familial, genetically transmitted disorder, but it has an inconsistent pattern of inheritance, including autosomal dominant, recessive, sex-linked, polygenic, and multifactorial patterns. The frequency of migraine in parents of probands ranges from 50 to 90%, increasing as the ascertainment method becomes more direct. In the only study that directly interviewed parents of migraineurs, 91% had a history of migraine that met the IHS criteria, whereas only a 56% parental history was obtained when probands were asked to comment on their own parents' history of migraine.[1] Twin studies have shown a higher concordance for migraine in monozygotic twins (mean 50%) than in dizygotic twins (mean 14%).[2] In one study, twins separated at birth and reared separately not only had a high concordance for migraine but also developed migraine at similar ages.[3] Twin studies suggest a strong genetic component for migraine, but a simple inheritance pattern has not been identified. Familial hemiplegic migraine is the first migraine syndrome found to be due to multiple distinct mutations on different chromosomes.

Familial hemiplegic migraine

Familial hemiplegic migraine is an autosomal dominant, genetically heterogeneous form of migraine with aura, with variable penetrance. The syndrome includes attacks of migraine without aura, migraine with typical aura, and severe episodes with prolonged aura (characterized by motor weakness that can last several days or weeks). Fever, meningismus, and impaired consciousness, ranging from confusion to profound coma, can also occur in association with the motor weakness. Headache may precede the hemiparesis, start during the weakness, or be absent altogether. The onset of the hemiparesis may be abrupt and simulate a stroke.[4] In a study by Bradshaw and Parsons,[5] all FHM patients had associated paresthesias; 88% had visual auras and 44% had speech disturbances. Weakness lasted less than 1 hour in 58% of patients; however, it lasted 1–3 hours in 14%, 3–24 hours in 12%, and between 1 day and 1 week in 16% of patients. The syndrome can change in an affected individual over his or her lifetime. A person who has FHM in adolescence may develop migraine with aura as an adult and migraine without aura later in life.[6]

The IHS has subdivided hemiplegic migraine into sporadic and familial forms (Table 4.1), both of which typically begin in childhood and cease with adulthood. The age of onset of hemiplegic migraine may be earlier than that of migraine without aura. The attacks themselves are frequently precipitated by minor head injury. Changes in consciousness ranging from confusion to coma are a feature, especially in childhood, and occurred in 23% of Bradshaw and Parsons' series.[5] The prevalence of hemiplegic migraine is uncertain and varies from 4 to 30%.[4,7] The differential diagnosis of hemiplegic migraine includes focal seizures, stroke, coagulopathies, CADASIL, and MELAS.

The headache of FHM can be generalized (29%), contralateral (47%), or ipsilateral (22%) to the hemiparesis. Before assessment, 17% of Bradshaw and Parsons'[5] patients had a single neurologic episode, 37% had between two and six episodes, and the remainder had more than seven attacks. The longer-lasting episodes were associated with more profound weakness and tended to be less frequent in their recurrence.

In 20% of unselected FHM families, patients can have fixed cerebellar symptoms and signs such as nystagmus and progressive ataxia. Cerebellar ataxia may occur before the first hemiplegic migraine attack and progress independent of the frequency or severity of the attacks. All these families have been shown to be linked to chromosome 19.[8]

Table 4.1. Familial hemiplegic migraine (IHS criteria).

Description:
   Migraine with aura including hemiparesis and where at least one
   first degree relative has identical attacks.

Diagnostic criteria:
   A. Fulfills criteria for 1.2 (migraine with aura).
   B. The aura includes some degree of hemiparesis and may be prolonged.
   At least one first degree relative has identical attacks.

In 1996, a Dutch group reported the first ever migraine genetic mutation in five families with FHM.[9] They identified, on chromosome 19p, four missense mutations in the CACNL1A4 gene, which encodes for the alpha1A subunit of a neuronal P/Q type voltage gated calcium channel. The P/Q type calcium channel regulates the release of specific neurotransmitters such as glutamate, dopamine, and possibly serotonin. They are found extensively in the brain, especially in the cerebellum, which explains the cerebellar symptoms in a subgroup of FHM patients. The alpha subunit of the P/Q calcium channel makes up the ion pore of the channel, thus determining the voltage and ion selectivity of the channel. The identified missense mutation on chromosome 19 appears to involve the transmembrane-spanning segments of the alpha1A subunit that form either the ion pore or voltage sensor (Fig. 4.1). The mutations may lead to a decrement in calcium passage through the channel with subsequent impairment in neurotransmitter release resulting in prolonged auras and migraine. Two other well-defined neurologic syndromes result from mutations in the CACNL1A4 gene include episodic ataxia type 2 and spinocerebellar ataxia type 6.

In 1997, a new genetic locus for FHM was identified by Gardner et al.[10] on chromosome 1q31 in a large family from Wyoming. These patients experienced a significant number of attacks of hemisensory loss along with hemiplegia. Attacks were triggered by mild head trauma in 83%. Ducros et al.[11] also reported another FHM mutation in three families from France on chromosome 1q21-23. The gene mutations on chromosome 1 have yet to be defined, but may involve a calcium or potassium channel. Several members in the chromosome 1q21-23 families developed seizures. Chromosome 1 FHM families differ from chromosome 19 families: some chromosome 1 family patients have seizures, while some chromosome 19 families have cerebellar ataxia.

CADASIL

Cerebral autosomal dominant arteriopathy with subcortical infarcts and leukoencephalopathy (CADASIL) is a rare, inherited neurodegenerative disorder recently mapped to chromosome 19q12.[12] It was formerly called hereditary multi-infarct dementia. It has been reported in more than 200 families worldwide.[13] The genetic defect involves the Notch3 gene, which codes for transmembrane receptor proteins. The syndrome usually presents with migraine with aura in the third decade, stroke-like spells in the fourth decade, and subcortical dementia with associated pseudobulbar palsy in the fifth decade, which occurs in one-third of affected family members and 90% of subjects before death. Affective disorders are a common part of the syndrome, occurring in 20% of sufferers. Death normally occurs by the sixth decade. Migraine with aura is the most common presenting symptom of CADASIL, occurring in 40% of subjects.[14] The mean age of onset of migraine in CADASIL

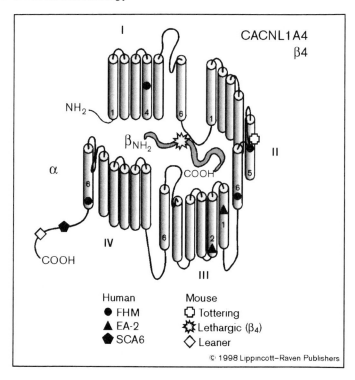

Fig. 4.1. Human and mouse mutations/disorders of calcium channel subunits CACNL1A4 and β4. The symbols indicate the relative positions of the different mutations in human familial hemiplegic migraine (FHM), episodic ataxia-2 (EA-2), spinocerebellar ataxia (SCA-6) and mouse disorders, *totterer*, *leaner*, and *lethargic*. There are six transmembrane segments making up the four domains of the CACNL1A4 P/Q calcium channel α subunit. The position of the β regularity β4 subunit and mutation in *lethargic* mice is shown relative to the α subunit.

patients is 30 years. Lacunar syndromes are the most common stroke type, occurring in 75% of patients.

Neuroimaging has played a pivotal role in the study of CADASIL. Magnetic resonance imaging findings are very suggestive of the diagnosis in the appropriate clinical setting. Characteristic MRI abnormalities can be detected before the appearance of symptoms, and can be used to diagnose CADASIL in genetically at-risk family members who have a pattern of autosomal dominant inheritance.[15]

Chabriat et al.[16] studied seven families with CADASIL and found that 50% of subjects aged 30–40 years had an abnormal computed tomography or MRI scan, while only 25% of them had symptoms of the disease. In the asymptomatic individuals, neuroimaging was diagnostic and not an adjunct procedure. Two main MRI abnormalities are observed in

CADASIL: (1) Extensive symmetric white matter abnormalities involving both periventricular and lobar white matter with a preponderance in the anterior temporal regions. There is absence of cortical lesions, sparing of the subcortical U fibers, and preference for the external capsule over the internal capsule. (2) Small, well-delineated, deep lesions with decreased signal on T1-weighted images and increased signal on T2-weighted images, consistent with lacunar infarctions involving the basal ganglia and thalamus.

The arteriopathy underlying the disorder is neither atherosclerotic nor amyloid and involves the media of small cerebral arteries. Lesions may also be found in extracerebral arteries, including skin arterioles. Ultrastructural examination reveals abnormal patches of agranular osmiophilic material within the basal membranes of vascular smooth-muscle cells.[17] A skin biopsy can be diagnostic.

Joutel et al.[13] identified Notch3 as the defective gene in CADASIL. Members of the Notch gene family encode evolutionarily conserved transmembrane receptors and are involved in cell fate specification during embryonic development. The Notch3 gene includes 33 exons encoding a protein of 2321 amino acids. Its extracellular domain contains 34 epidermal growth factor-like repeats. From data on *Drosophila*, this extracellular domain seems to be involved in ligand-binding, whereas the intracellular domain carries the intrinsic signal-transducing activity. CADASIL gene identification provided the basic information needed to set up a direct genotypic diagnostic test.[17]

Fifty unrelated patients with CADASIL and 100 healthy controls were screened for mutations along the entire Notch3 sequence by means of single-strand conformation polymorphism, heteroduplex, and sequence analysis. Strongly stereotyped missense mutations, located within the epidermal growth factor-like repeats in the extracellular domain of Notch3, were detected in 45 of the CADASIL patients. Clustering of mutations within the two exons encoding the first five epidermal growth factor-like repeats was observed in 32 patients. All these mutations lead to loss or gain of a cysteine residue and therefore to an unpaired number of cysteine residues within a given epidermal growth factor-like domain. None of these mutations was found in the 100 controls.[13]

Disorders that can potentially be confused with CADASIL on MRI include Binswangers disease, metachromatic leukodystrophy, subacute sclerosing panencephalitis, multiple sclerosis, and progressive multifocal leukoencephalopathy. These disorders, however, lack the dominating history of migraine headache. FHM is distinguished from CADASIL by its earlier onset, benign prognosis, and normal imaging findings.

MELAS

Mitochondrial encephalomyopathy, lactic acidosis, and stroke-like spells (MELAS) is a mitochondrial inherited disease in which 50–80% of sufferers have migraine. In most individuals, the onset of stroke, seizures, and lactic acidosis occurs before age 40. Headache (usually migraine), seizures, and gastrointestinal symptoms (nausea, vomiting) are the most common presenting symptoms of MELAS. MELAS was the first clue that there was a connection between mitochondrial function and migraine. Many patients with MELAS were said to have 'malignant migraine' prior to the identification of their mitochondrial defect.[18]

At first MELAS patients are neurologically intact, but they later develop focal neurologic abnormalities, typically a visual field deficit or hemiparesis. When the disease begins before age 20, about 30% of patients die before age 30.[19]

Hirano and Pavlakis[19] reviewed 110 documented cases of MELAS. Computed tomographic examinations showed cortical infarction in 80% of imaged patients. The infarcts were present in the occipital, parietal, and temporal lobes and some resolved (on follow-up scans) in hours to days. Cortical atrophy occurred in about 30% of MELAS patients and basal ganglia calcifications in 43%. MELAS infarcts are felt to be metabolically induced and nonvascular, as they frequently do not respect arterial boundaries and their disappearance within days of the initial event can be documented with neuroimaging. One explanation for MELAS-induced strokes is an angiopathy caused by mitochondrial-induced defects of endothelial cells and smooth muscle cells of blood vessels.[20] Another hypothesis is that oxidative phosphorylation defects lead to oxygen free radical production, with resultant neutralization of vasodilators such as nitrous oxide, thus leading to reflex vasoconstriction and stroke.[21]

Three major mtDNA point mutations have been identified in MELAS patients. The most common, found in 80–90% of patients, is an A-to-G transition at nucleotide 3243 of tRNALeu(UUR). Less common is a T-to-C transition at nucleotide 3271, which occurs in 7.5% of patients; one rare ND4 mutation (subunit 4 of complex I) has been identified. Nuclear DNA mutations can cause MELAS, but this is rare.

What is the connection between migraine, which is a very common medical condition that affects 10% of the population, and mitochondrial disorders, which are rare? Both migraine and MELAS are associated primarily with posterior circulation strokes.[22] Maternal inheritance, the pattern found with mtDNA mutations, is well documented in migraineurs. Not all individuals in migraine families have migraine, and migraine, if it occurs, may begin at different ages and present with varying severities in different family members. This is similar to what is seen in families with mtDNA-based disorders. Due to heteroplasmy and the threshold effect, different family members have varying amounts of abnormal mtDNA and, depending on the amount, may have a full-blown multisystem mitochondrial disorder or may be asymptomatic or oligosymptomatic. Relatives of patients with MELAS syndrome may suffer with migraine headaches only.

Migraine may be due to mitochondrial dysfunction in some patients.

Sachs et al.[23] found a reduced cerebral metabolic rate of glucose metabolism measured by positron emission tomography scanning in migraineurs (both with and without aura) who had been given reserpine. Bousser et al.[24] and Sigrid et al.[25] found increased cerebral oxygen consumption in migraineurs with aura. Metabolic studies in migraineurs that specifically suggest mitochondrial dysfunction include elevated cerebrospinal fluid lactate levels during headaches, platelet hyposecretion of adenosine 5′-triphosphate (ATP),[26] and baseline elevated serum lactate and pyruvate levels compared with controls.[27]

Montagna et al.[28] tested markers of mitochondrial metabolism in nine women migraineurs (four had prolonged aura and five had stroke occurring during an episode of migraine) who ranged in age from 16 to 48 years. None had any identified cardiovascular risk factors for stroke, and cerebral angiography was normal in eight of the women. Resting venous lactate levels were no different from 10 age-matched controls. However, lactate levels during exertion were disproportionately higher in the migraineurs compared with the control subjects. In eight patients, platelet NADH-cytochrome-c-reductase levels (Complexes I and III of the electron transport chain) were significantly lower than in controls. Muscle mitochondrial enzyme activity showed a mean reduction of 37% for NADH-cytochrome-c-reductase activity, 30% for cytochrome oxidase, 27% for succinate-cytochrome-c-reductase, 22% for NADH dehydrogenase, and 16% for succinate dehydrogenase, while citrate synthase levels were within the normal range. The changes were restricted to enzymes of the electron transport chain, as citrate synthase resides in the mitochondrial matrix. One patient with migrainous stroke had ragged-red fibers on muscle biopsy; the remainder of the patients had normal muscle histology.

Sangiorgi et al.[29] analyzed platelet mitochondrial enzymes in 40 patients with migraine without aura, 40 patients with migraine with aura (between attacks), and 24 controls. In both migraine subgroups, NADH-dehydrogenase (Complex I), cytochrome c-oxidase (Complex IV), and citrate synthase (Krebs cycle) levels were reduced compared with controls. NADH-cytochrome-reductase activity (Complex I and III) was slightly low only in migraineurs with aura. They concluded that a general impairment of energy metabolism and a systemic defect in mitochondrial function exists in migraineurs. This, though, was probably not secondary to mutations in mtDNA, as citrate synthase is encoded by nuclear DNA and maternal transmission was not identified in their patient population.

Mitochondrial DNA mutations have been demonstrated in migraineurs. Bresolin et al.[30] identified a DNA deletion without the A-to-G point mutation at nucleotide 3243 in the mitochondrial tRNA[LEU] gene (the MELAS mutation) in a patient with recurrent migraine-related strokes. The patient had no evidence of muscle weakness or atrophy, but muscle biopsy revealed ragged-red and cytochrome-c-oxidase negative fibers. Mosewich et al.[31] reported on a large family with the tRNA[LEU] point mutation at position 3243, which is specific for MELAS. Most members of the family never had a stroke but did have frequent migraine attacks. Ojaimi et al.[32] screened for mtDNA mutations in patients presenting with thrombotic stroke and a history of migraine with aura. Primary mutations associated with MELAS and Leber's hereditary optic neuropathy were not detected, but they did identify increased levels of two secondary Leber's hereditary optic neuropathy mutations. The G-to-A mutation at 13 708 and the T-to-C mutation at nucleotide 4216 were more common than expected.

Klopstock et al.[22] completed the largest mtDNA study in migraineurs, analyzing lymphocytic mtDNA in 23 patients with migraine with aura using the polymerase chain reaction and southern blot analysis. They screened for point mutations at base pair 3243 (MELAS) and base pair 8344 (MERF) and for large-scale deletions. No deletions or point mutations were identified at these sites. The study could not exclude the presence of other mtDNA mutations or nuclear coded mutations for respiratory chain subunits in the migraineurs who were studied. At the time of writing no specific mtDNA mutation has been identified that links to any subsets of migraine patients.

Magnetic resonance spectroscopy (MRS) has helped to clarify the relationship between migraine and mitochondrial energy metabolism. Using phosphorus MRS (^{31}P-MRS), one can estimate levels of phosphocreatinine (PCr, measure of high energy phosphates), inorganic phosphate (Pi, measure of low energy phosphate states), ADP, intracellular pHi, and intracellular magnesium concentrations. Muscle MRS can measure post-exercise recovery of PCr, which is a direct measure of mitochondrial function since PCr resynthesis is entirely dependent on mitochondrial respiration.[33]

Welch et al.[34] compared cortical energy metabolism in a group of migraineurs with and without aura with control subjects. Migraineurs, during attacks, had a loss of high energy phosphates and an elevation of low energy phosphates, suggesting that energy phosphate metabolism is altered in migraineurs during attacks and that migraine initiation may be secondary to cortical energy failure.[34]

Montagna et al.[35] carried out three separate investigations using ^{31}P-MRS, examining three separate migraine subclasses in between attacks. The initial study looked at 15 patients with complicated migraine (migraine with prolonged aura and migrainous stroke).[36] The other two investigations looked at 12 migraineurs with aura[37] and 22 migraineurs without aura, respectively.[35] Brain ^{31}P-MRS was abnormal in all migraine subtypes (there was an interictal loss of high energy phosphates), indicating an unstable metabolic state in the brain cells of migraineurs between migraine attacks.

Muscle MRS, looking for recovery of PCr, was abnormal in all complicated migraine patients and delayed in 13 of 18 patients with aura and 12 of 22 patients without aura. Migraineurs appear to have a fixed defect in energy metabolism independent of the migraine attack. This abnormal energy metabolism is present in all migraine subtypes and may be due to mitochondrial dysfunction. The abnormalities are not exclusive to the brain and extend to tissue outside the CNS.

Riboflavin, a precursor of flavin nucleotides, has recently been shown to be an effective migraine preventive agent in one placebo-controlled trial, further strengthening the relationship between migraine and mitochondrial function.[38]

Treatment

Treatment for FHM or migraine with prolonged aura has not been studied in controlled trials. Most experts treat FHM patients preventively with calcium channel blockers. Verapamil appears to reduce the frequency and severity of the prolonged motor aura spells. The mechanism is unknown. Perhaps they are correcting an abnormal calcium channel or preventing arterial vasospasm that leads to decreased cortical blood flow and thus the neurologic symptoms of the migraine aura. Both single photon emission computed tomography (SPECT) and functional MR imaging have demonstrated a reduced cortical cerebral blood flow during aura.[39,40] Transcranial Doppler studies suggest this hypoperfusion may be caused by arterial vasospasm.[41] Some experts suggest that patients with FHM or prolonged auras should not be treated with beta blockers because of the belief that these agents may add to the stroke risks in this patient population.

Flunarizine, a calcium channel blocker not available in the USA, has proven efficacy for migraine prevention in both children and adults. Flunarizine may be especially useful in the treatment of FHM, as it has been shown to increase the threshold for cortical spreading depression (the neurophysiologic event believed to cause human aura).[42]

Divalproex sodium is an FDA-approved migraine preventive drug. Its action in preventing migraine probably relates to its ability to enhance the action of GABA. In addition, it is an effective treatment for migraine with persistent aura.[43] Some experts use low-dose aspirin to decrease both attack frequency and stroke risk.

Acute headache treatment of FHM patients is limited. Many experts believe that vasoconstrictive drugs such as triptans, ergots, or dihydroergotamine should not be used. Some believe that these agents would increase the stroke risk in these patients. Treatments to abort prolonged auras include inhalation of 10% carbon dioxide (in 90% oxygen), amyl nitrate, and isoproterenol, but all have been in uncontrolled studies and the results have been mixed.[44] In our opinion, dopamine receptor antagonists (e.g. i.v. or p.r. prochlorperazine) are useful in controlling prolonged auras. Patients with FHM and prolonged auras should have access to prochlorperazine suppositories, because they will usually abort an attack if they are utilized early. Migraine with aura is associated with a variation in the DRD2 gene, and both the aura and the migraine headache may be generated by a hyperdopaminergic state.[45] Intravenous magnesium can be used alone or in combination with intravenous neuroleptics to break prolonged auras.

The migraine aura is believed to be caused by cortical spreading depression (CSD). In vitro, glutamate-induced spreading depression can be inhibited by magnesium, suggesting that magnesium should alleviate CSD-induced auras in humans.[46]

Diagnosis

Familial hemiplegic migraine.

References

1. Devoto M, Lozito A, Staffa G et al. Segregation analysis of migraine in 128 families. *Cephalalgia* 1986; **6:** 101–105.
2. Haan J, Terwindt GM, Ferrari MD. Genetics of migraine. In: Mathew NT, ed. *Advances in Headache. Neurol Clin* 1997; **15:** 43–60.
3. Juel-Nielsen N. Individual and environment: a psychiatric investigation of monozygotic twins reared apart. *Acta Psychiatr Scand* 1964, **40:** 1–251.
4. Whitty CWM. Familial hemiplegic migraine. In: Rose FC, ed. *Handbook of Clinical Neurology*. Amsterdam: Elsevier, 1986: 141–153.
5. Bradshaw P, Parsons M. Hemiplegic migraine, a clinical study. *Q J Med* 1965; **133:** 65–85.
6. Stewart WF, Shechter AL, Lipton RB. Migraine heterogeneity: disability, pain intensity, attack frequency, and duration. *Neurology* 1994; **44:** S24–S39.
7. Selby G, Lance JW. Observation on 500 cases of migraine and allied vascular headaches. *J Neurol Neurosurg Psychiatry* 1960; **23:** 23–32.
8. Tournier-Lasserve E. Hemiplegic migraine, episodic ataxia type 2: and the others. *Neurology* 1999; **53:** 3–4.
9. Ophoff RA, Terwindt GM, Vergouwe MN. Familial hemiplegic migraine and episodic ataxia type-2 are caused by mutations in the Ca^{2+} channel gene CACNLA4. *Cell Tiss Res* 1996; **87:** 543–552.
10. Gardner K, Barmada MM, Patek LJ et al. A new locus for hemiplegic migraine maps to chromosome 1q31. *Neurology* 1997; **49:** 1231–1238.
11. Ducros A, Joutel A, Vahedi, K. Mapping of a second locus for familial hemiplegic migraine to 1q21-q23 and evidence of further heterogeneity. *Ann Neurol* 1997; **42:** 885–890.
12. Bousser MG, Tournier-Lasserve E 1994. Summary of the proceedings of the first international workshop on CADASIL, Paris, May 19–21. *Stroke*, **25:** 704–707.
13. Joutel A, Corpechot C, Ducros A et al. Notch3 mutations in CADASIL, a hereditary adult-onset condition causing stroke and dementia. *Nature* 1996; **383:** 707–710.
14. Dichgans M, Mayer M, Uttner I et al. The phenotypic spectrum of CADASIL: clinical findings in 102 cases. *Ann Neurol* 1998; **44:** 731–739.
15. Hutchinson M, O'Riordan J, Javed M et al. Familial hemiplegic migraine and autosomal dominant arteriopathy with leukoencephalopathy. *Ann Neurol* 1995; **38:** 817–824.

16. Chabriat H, Vahedi K, Iba-Zizen MT et al. 1995. Clinical spectrum of CADASIL: a study of seven families. *Lancet*; **346**: 934–939.
17. Joutel A, Vahedi K, Corpechot C et al. Strong clustering and stereotyped nature of Notch3 mutations in CADASIL patients. *Lancet* 1997; **350**: 1511–1515.
18. Andermann, F, Lugaresi, E, Dvorkin, GS et al. Malignant migraine: the syndrome of prolonged classical migraine, epilepsia partialis continua, and repeated strokes: a clinically characteristic disorder probably due to mitochondrial encephalopathy. *Funct Neurol* 1986; **1**: 481–486.
19. Hirano M, Pavlakis SG. Mitochondrial myopathy, encephalopathy, lactic acidosis, and stroke-like episodes (MELAS): current concepts. *J Child Neurol* 1994; **9**: 4–13.
20. Ohama E, Ohara S, Ikuta F et al. Mitochondrial angiopathy in the cerebral blood vessels of MELAS (mitochondrial myopathy, encephalopathy, lactic acidosis, and stroke-like episodes). *Brain Nerve* 1988; **40**: 109–118.
21. Luft R, Landua BR. Mitochondrial medicine. *J Intern Med* 1995; **238**: 405–421.
22. Klopstock T, May A, Seibel P et al. Mitochondrial DNA in migraine with aura. *Neurology* 1996; **46**: 1735–1738.
23. Sachs H, Wolf A, Russell JA et al. Effects of reserpine on regional cerebral glucose metabolism in control and migraine subjects. *Arch Neurol* 1986; **43**: 1117–1123.
24. Bousser MG, Baron JC, Iba-Zizen MT et al. Migrainous cerebral infarction; a tomographic study of cerebral blood flow and oxygen extraction fraction with the oxygen-15 inhalation technique. *Stroke* 1980; **148**: 145–53.
25. Sigrid H, Gibbs JM, Jones AD et al. Oxygen metabolism in migraine. *J Cereb Blood Flow Metab* 1985; **5**: S445–S446.
26. Joseph R, Welch KMA, D'Andrea G et al. ATP hyposecretion from platelet dense bodies – evidence for the purigenic hypothesis and a marker of migraine. *Headache* 1986; **26**: 403–410.
27. Okada H, Araga S, Takeshima T et al. Plasma lactic acid and pyruvic acid levels in migraine and tension-type headache. *Headache* 1998; **38**: 39–42.
28. Montagna P, Sacquegna T, Martinelli P et al. Mitochondrial abnormalities in migraine: preliminary findings. *Headache* 1988; **28**: 477–480.
29. Sangiorgi S, Mochi M, Riva R et al. Abnormal platelet mitochondrial function in patients affected by migraine with and without aura. *Cephalalgia* 1994; **14**: 21–23.
30. Bresolin N, Martinelli P, Barbiroli B et al. Muscle mitochondrial deletion and ^{31}P-NMR spectroscopy alterations in a migraine patient. *J Neurol Sci* 1991; **104**: 182–189.
31. Mosewich RK, Donat JR, DiMauro S et al. The syndrome of mitochondrial encephalomyopathy, lactic acidosis, and stroke-like episodes presenting without stroke. *Arch Neurol* 1993; **50**: 275–278.
32. Ojaimi J, Katsabanis S, Bower S et al. Mitochondrial DNA in stroke and migraine with aura. *Cerebrovasc Dis* 1998; **8**: 102–106.
33. Taylor DJ, Bore PJ, Styles P et al. Bioenergetics of intact human muscle: a ^{31}P nuclear magnetic resonance study. *Mol Bio Med* 1983; **1**: 77–94.
34. Welch KMA, Levine SRDG, Schultz L et al. Preliminary observations on brain energy metabolism in migraine studied by in vivo 31-phosphorus NMR spectroscopy. *Neurology* 1989 **39**: 538–541.

35. Montagna P, Cortelli P, Monari L et al. ^{31}P-Magnetic resonance spectroscopy in migraine without aura. *Neurology* 1994; **44:** 666–668.
36. Barbiroli B, Montagna P, Cortelli P et al. Complicated migraine studied by phosphorus magnetic resonance spectroscopy. *Cephalalgia* 1990; **10:** 263–272.
37. Barbiroli B, Montagna P, Cortelli P. et al. Abnormal brain and muscle energy metabolism shown by 31P magnetic resonance spectroscopy in patients affected by migraine with aura. *Neurology* 1992; **42:** 1209–1214.
38. Schoenen J, Jacquy J, Lenaerts M. Effectiveness of high-dose riboflavin in migraine prophylaxis. A randomized controlled trial. *Neurology* 1998; **50:** 466–470.
39. Andersen AR, Friberg L, Skyloj-Olsen T et al. Delayed hyperemia following hypoperfusion in classic migraine. Single photon emission tomographic demonstration. *Arch Neurol* 1988; **45:** 154–159.
40. Cutrer FM, Sorenson AG, Weisskoff RM et al. Perfusion-weighted imaging defects during spontaneous migrainous aura. *Ann Neurol* 1998; **43:** 25–31.
41. Totaro R, DeMatteis G, Marini C et al. Cerebral blood flow in migraine with aura: a transcranial sonography study. *Headache* 1992; **32:** 446–51.
42. Wauquier A, Ashton D, Marranes R. The effects of flunarizine in experimental models related to the pathogenesis of migraine. *Cephalalgia* 1985; **5:** 119–120.
43. Rothrock JF. Successful treatment of persistent migraine aura with divalproex sodium. *Neurology* 1997; **27:** 484–486.
44. Silberstein SD, Young WB. Migraine aura and prodrome. *Semin Neurol* 1995; **45:** 175–182.
45. Peroutka SJ, Wilhoit T, Jones K. Clinical susceptibility to migraine with aura is modified by dopamine D2 receptor (DRD2) NcoI alleles. *Neurology* 1997; **49:** 201–206.
46. Van Harreveld A. Two mechanisms for spreading depression in the chicken retina. *J Neurobiol* 1978; **9:** 419–431.

5

Progressive ataxia and dysarthria

Clinical history and examination

A 56-year-old, right-handed physician had noted progressive gait impairment and dysarthria for 1 year, but he had no tremor, oscillopsia, tendency to fall, bladder symptoms or fainting episodes. Anxiety and shortness of breath were other symptoms. He was a practicing gastroenterologist and was otherwise in good health. His medications included Elavil 50 mg, and Mevacor 20 mg daily.

Family history: His brother, age 54 years, also had dysarthria and gait ataxia. His brother drank alcohol excessively. No other members were known to be similarly affected. His mother lived to age 78 with progressive dementia. The maternal great grandmother had a gait disorder that was not well characterized. Three other siblings were neurologically intact, as were his five children.

Examination: Blood pressure, 110/70; pulse, 92; weight, 172 lbs. He appeared to be in no acute distress. Findings on general physical examination were unremarkable. His chest was clear to auscultation; heart rhythm and sounds were normal. The abdomen was unremarkable. His extremities showed no abnormalities.

He was alert, oriented and had normal language function. Visual acuity was 20/20 with glasses; the pupils were equal and reacted to light and accommodation. Ocular movements were full, with no nystagmus on lateral or vertical gaze. The optic fundi showed slight pallor of the discs. Facial sensation and facial muscle strength were normal. Lingual and pharyngeal functions were also normal, including the gag reflex. His speech had a scanning quality and was markedly dysarthric. Muscle bulk, tone, and strength were normal, as were the tendon reflexes and plantar responses. His finger-to-nose and heel-to-shin tests demonstrated dysmetria and ataxia. There were no involuntary movements or tremor. His gait was broad based and ataxic; he could not walk tandem. Sensation for all modalities was normal.

Laboratory data: The following blood tests gave normal results: blood glucose, urea nitrogen, creatinine, electrolytes, calcium, phosphorus, total protein, alkaline phosphatase, bilirubin, lactate dehydrogenase, creatine kinase. Thyroid functions were normal. Erythrocyte sedimentation rate, complete blood count and anti-nuclear antibody studies were normal. Serum cholesterol was 228 mg/dl. Brain MRI (Fig. 5.1) showed a persistent cavum septum pellucidum and evidence of atrophy of the cerebellum involving the hemispheres and the vermis.

Course: In the next 2 years, there was progression of dysarthria, dysmetria, impaired coordination of his limbs and gait ataxia. He used a cane or a walker for walking. His younger brother also noted progression of dysarthria and gait ataxia. A diagnostic test was obtained.

$$* \quad * \quad *$$

Discussion

For 2 years, this 56-year-old physician had a progressive ataxia and dysarthria as did his younger brother. His intellectual functions remained normal. Eye movements were also normal and he had no nystagmus. There were no abnormalities of sensation and there were no upper or lower motor neuron signs. At first it was thought the brother may have had an alcoholic cerebellar degeneration. He declined further medical evaluation. There was no evidence of multiple sclerosis, hypothyroidism, abetalipoproteinemia, or malignant tumor.

Both the patient and the brother showed symmetrical impairment of cerebellar functions, beginning rather late in life and without intellectual impairment, visual loss, abnormal cranial nerve functions, or abnormal pyramidal or extrapyramidal motor functions.

Brain MRI showed no evidence of mass effect, demyelinating disease, infarcts, microvascular changes or cerebral atrophy. It did show cerebellar atrophy affecting the hemispheres and vermis.

Thus the patient had a familial cerebellar degeneration. The pedigree was incomplete and did not suffice to determine if inheritance was autosomal dominant or autosomal recessive. Neurological symptoms in the mother and maternal great grandmother suggested autosomal dominant inheritance. Although the mother showed dementia, the patient remained intellectually intact, making Huntington disease unlikely. Ataxia is sometimes the first symptom of Huntington disease but this patient had no chorea. Dementia in the mother, motor abnormality in the great grandmother, and ataxia in two brothers in the most recent generation raise the possibility of Gerstman–Straussler–Schenker disease. This is an autosomal dominant prion disease resulting from a mutation in the prion gene on chromosome 20 involving codon 102. Again, this diversity of presentation and the lack of mental alterations in the propositus makes that disorder highly unlikely.

The most likely diagnosis was a familial spinocerebellar ataxia. Spinocerebellar ataxias 1–11 (SCA-1–11) have been mapped to different chromosomal locations.[1-8] SCA-1 maps to chromosome 6p22-p23 and is caused by unstable expanded CAG repeats in a coding region of the SCA-1 gene.[9] The gene product, ataxin 1, has not been characterized. Up to 36 CAGs are normal, patients have 38 CAGs or more. Anticipation is evident, with an increased number of CAG unstable DNA triplet repeats in the next generation, earlier age at onset, and more severe disabilities. Signs include ophthalmoparesis, nystagmus, myokymia of periorbital and perioral muscles, and dysarthria. Gait ataxia is an early and dominant feature with progressive hyperreflexia, clonus and extensor plantar responses in many patients. There may be some intellectual decline. Pyramidal and extrapyramidal features with dystonia are seen with higher numbers of CAG repeats. Our patient conformed to late onset SCA-1 with a purely cerebellar disorder.

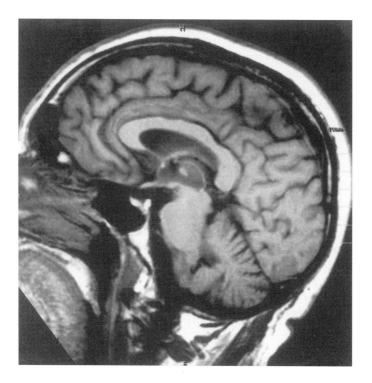

Fig. 5.1. Sagittal MRI of the brain of a 60-year-man with gait ataxia and dysarthria. Cerebellar and brainstem atrophy are evident.

SCA-2 maps to 12q23-q24.1 and is also due to CAG unstable repeats.[8] It was first described in families from Cuba with an autosomal dominant pattern of ataxia, slow saccadic eye movements, and areflexia. Some patients show reflexes and dystonia. The mutant protein, ataxin-2, has not been characterized. The normal number of CAG repeats is 15–24; affected individuals show 35–59 repeats and anticipation has been described.

The patient could have had Machado–Joseph disease (MJD) or SCA-3, an autosomal dominant spinocerebellar degenerative disorder that was first described among the Portuguese and their descendants in the USA and Brazil. It occurs worldwide and is the most common inherited autosomal dominant ataxia. It maps to 14q24.3-q32; normal individuals have 12–37 CAG repeats and patients between 60 and 84 CAG repeats.[8,10] The mutant protein, MJD-ataxin, has not been characterized but it is one of the polyglutamine-containing proteins corresponding to the CAG codon for glutamine.[8,10,11] Symptoms may begin in childhood with impressive spasticity and dystonia. If the onset is in adolescence or early adult years, findings include true ataxia, spasticity and dystonia. Onset after age 50 may be manifest by a pure cerebellar syndrome and amyotrophy. A syndrome of parkinsonism, ataxia and amyotrophy has also been described. The findings in our patient were consistent with late-onset form of MJD.

SCA-4 is another autosomal dominant disorder that maps to 16q24-tER; manifestations include prominent axonal neuropathy and ataxia, which was not the combination in our patient.[8]

SCA-5, a late-onset cerebellar degeneration, maps to chromosome 11. Families have been traced back to two branches of descendants of President Abraham Lincoln.[8]

SCA-6 is another late onset cerebellar degeneration. It involves the gene for the P/Q (1A voltage calcium channel subunit, which maps to chromosome 19p13. Normal individuals have 4–16 CAG repeats. Patients have 21–27 repeats and signs of late-onset progressive cerebellar degeneration. Allelic mutations are either missense or nonsense mutations. The missense mutations result in familial hemiplegic migraine; the nonsense mutations result in premature termination of synthesis of the gene product with hereditary paroxysmal ataxia and hemiplegia in some patients. Our patient with a CAG expansion had late onset ataxia.[8,12–14]

SCA-7 is also an autosomal dominant syndrome of progressive ataxia with a CAG expansion that maps to 3p14.1-p21.1. The patient here did not have macular degeneration or pigmentary retinal degeneration, making SCA-7 unlikely.[8,15]

SCA-8 comprises nystagmus, spastic paraparesis and reduced vibratory sensation mapping to 13q21. The CTG expansion affects an untranslated region of the gene.[8,16]

SCA-10, also dominantly inherited, maps to 22q; in some patients the major manifestation is a seizure disorder.[8,17]

SCA-11 has been recognized in one British family, maps to 15q14-q21.3, and causes a pure cerebellar syndrome of mid-life.[8,12]

The patient here could have had SCA-1, MJD or SCA-6 to account for the late onset of a pure cerebellar syndrome of dysarthria, gait ataxia, and limb ataxia. Late-onset MJD can include progressive ataxia and dysarthria but is often associated with amyotrophy, which this patient lacked. SCA-6 is rare but the clinical syndrome and the cerebellar atrophy were compatible.

DNA testing was conducted for SCA-1 in one patient and his brother. The normal number of CAG repeats for SCA-1 is up to 36; patients show more than 36. The patient had 38 CAG repeats involving allele 1 and 30 CAG repeats in allele 2. His brother also had 38 CAG repeats in allele 1 and 23 CAG repeats in allele 2.[8,9] The molecular diagnosis of SCA-1 was established in this family with a modest but abnormal number of expanded repeats and a mild late-onset syndrome of a pure cerebellar disorder, without pyramidal or extrapyramidal features.

This family illustrates the need to ascertain the genotype of any dominantly inherited ataxia. The phenotype in this family corresponded nonspecifically to any of four disorders: SCA-1, MJD, SCA-5, and SCA-6. The genotype settled the issue. DNA analysis was essential in providing accurate neurological diagnosis and, particularly, genetic counseling for other family members.[8]

Diagnosis

Spinocerebellor ataxia (SCA)-1.

References

1. Conner KE, Rosenberg RN. The hereditary ataxias. In Rosenberg RN, Prusiner SB, DiMauro S, Barchi RL, eds. *The Molecular and Genetic Basis of Neurological Disease*, 2nd edn. Boston: Butterworth-Heinemann, 1997: 503–544.
2. Rosenberg RN. Autosomal dominant cerebellar phenotypes: the genotype has settled the issue. *Neurology* 1995; **45:** 1.
3. Rosenberg RN. DNA triplet repeats and neurologic disease. *N Engl J Med* 1996; **335:** 1222.
4. Rosenberg RN. The genetic basis of ataxia. *Clin Neurosci* 1995; **3:** 1.
5. Rosenberg RN. Spinocerebellar ataxias and ataxins. *N Engl J Med* 1995; **333:** 1351.
6. Rosenberg RN, Iannaccone ST. The prevention of neurogenetic disease. *Arch Neurol* 1995; **52:** 356.
7. Rosenberg RN, Iannaccone ST. Genetic neurological diseases. In: Rosenberg RN, Pleasure DE. *Comprehensive Neurology*. New York: John Wiley, 1998: 33–113.
8. Rosenberg RN. Ataxic disorders. In: Fauci AS, Braunwald E, Isselbacher KJ, Wilson JD, Martin JB, Kasper DL, Hauser SL, Longo DL, eds. *Harrison's Textbook of Medicine*, 15th edn. New York: McGraw-Hill, in press.

9. Orr HT et al. Expansion of an unstable trinucleotide CAG repeat in spinocerebellar ataxia type 1. *Nat Genet* 1993; **4:** 221.

10. Kawaguchi Y et al. CAG expansions in a novel gene for Machado–Joseph disease at chromosome 14q32.1. *Nat Genet* 1994; **8:** 221.

11. Paulson HL, Perez MK, Trottier Y et al. Intranuclear inclusions of expanded polyglutamine protein in spinocerebellar ataxia type 3. *Neuron* 1997; **19:** 333–344.

12. Worth PF, Guinti P, Gardner-Thorpe C et al. Autosomal dominant cerebellar ataxia Type III: linkage in a large British family to a 7.6cM region on chromosome 15q14-q21.3. *Am J Hum Genet* 1999; **65:** 420–426.

13. Zhuchenko O et al. Autosomal dominant cerebellar ataxia (SCA6) associated with small polyglutamine expansions in the a1A-voltage-dependent calcium channel. *Nat Genet* 1997; **15:** 62.

14. Zoghbi HY. CAG repeats in SCAG6. *Neurology* 1997; **49:** 1196–1199.

15. Holmberg M, Duyckaerts C, Dürr A et al. Spinocerebellar ataxia type 7 (SCA7): a neurodegenerative disorder with neuronal intranuclear inclusions. *Hum Mol Genet* 1998; **7:** 913–918.

16. Koob M, Mosely M, Schut L et al. An untranslated CTG expansion causes a novel form of spinocerebellar ataxia (SCA8). *Nat Genet* 1999; **121:** 379–384.

17. Matsuura T, Achari M, Khajavi B et al. Mapping of the gene for a novel spinocerebellar ataxia with pure cerebellar signs and epilepsy. *Ann Neurol* 1999; **45:** 407–411.

6

A clinically pure lower motor neuron syndrome

Clinical history and examination

In December 1995, at age 74, this man noted left foot-drop. In April 1996, EMG showed widespread denervation with normal conduction studies. Cerebrospinal fluid protein content was 66 mg/dl, with no oligoclonal bands or white blood cells. An IgG lambda monoclonal gammopathy was found. Bone marrow was normal and there were no bone lesions. He had no paresthesias, sphincter symptoms, rash or weight loss and cramps were rare. In November 1996, another neurologist found distal weakness in both legs and fasciculations were not evident. Tendon jerks were present except that the ankle jerks were absent. A nerve biopsy showed sparse regenerative clusters of small myelinated fibers; stains for amyloid gave negative results. He was treated with intravenous immuno-globulins (IVIGs) and cyclophosphamide (intravenously once a month) without benefit. By October 1997 his hands had become weak and he had lost 20 pounds. Past history and family history were otherwise unre-markable. He had been a varsity baseball player at a major university.

Examination of the cranial nerve functions was normal except for a snout reflex. There was no dysarthria or lingual fasciculation. There was slight weakness of proximal arm muscles. The hands were weak and wasted. The psoas muscles were weak against gravity on the left and against slight resistance on the right. The left quadriceps was weak against gravity but was barely affected on the right. Distal muscles were also more severely affected on the left. Tendon reflexes were feeble in the left arm and were not elicited on the right. The knee jerks were brisk but ankle jerks were not elicited. The great toe extensors were paralyzed so there were no Babinski signs but there was a response of the tensor fascia lata on both sides. There was no Hoffmann sign or clonus and fasciculations were not seen.

The clinical signs were those of lower motor neuron disease except for the brisk knee jerks and, perhaps, the snout reflex. MR spectroscopy of the motor cortex gave NAA/Cr (N-acetyl aspartate:creatine) ratios of 2.2 on the right and 2.1 on the left, both distinctly below the normal lower limit of 2.50.[1] If taken at face value this result would have made the diagnosis of amyotrophic lateral sclerosis (ALS), but experience at the time had been too meager to warrant that conclusion.

A month later, in November 1997, he stopped walking because his arms and hands were too weak to hold the aluminum walker. He needed help for dressing. Findings on examination had not changed much. Tendon jerks were absent in the arms and the knee jerks were still brisk. The monoclonal gammopathy persisted. IVIG therapy again gave no benefit. Nerve conduction studies again failed to show any abnormality. Riluzole and antioxidants were added to his regimen. By May 1998 he had had a tracheostomy and a gastrostomy. He died with aspiration pneumonia in June 1998, 2.5 years after the onset of leg weakness. Post-mortem examination was performed.

*   *   *

Discussion

This patient had a progressively debilitating and ultimately fatal disease that was characterized by weakness and wasting of muscle, without visible fasciculation. The distal weakness was more like a neurogenic disorder than a myopathy, which is more often proximal. However, that distinction cannot be made solely by the distribution of weakness because there are distal myopathies. The lack of visible fasciculation left open the neurogenic or myopathic nature of the disorder, which was therefore defined by the EMG. The lack of upper motor neuron signs differentiated it from amyotrophic lateral sclerosis itself. It was a purely lower motor neuron disorder.

A category of 'ALS with probable upper motor neuron signs', ALS-PUMNS, has been used by some students to include patients who have incongruously active tendon jerks in limbs with weak, wasted and fasciculating limbs. This has been taken as a combination almost pathognomonic of ALS, but that is no longer true, as we discuss later. This patient had active knee jerks and a snout reflex, but these were not deemed sufficient to qualify for ALS-PUMNS.

In 1994,[2] ALS experts met in El Escorial, Spain, to define criteria for the diagnosis of ALS so that patients entering therapeutic trials would be reasonably homogeneous in expression of the disease. According to those criteria, 'definite' ALS is diagnosed when there are both upper and lower motor neuron signs in three body regions, including the head. 'Probable' ALS is the term used if both upper motor neuron and lower motor neuron signs are present in two body regions, and 'possible' if only one body region shows both sets of signs. If, as in this patient, there are only lower motor neuron signs, the condition is only 'suspected.'

There are three possible diagnoses:

First, he could have had *adult-onset progressive spinal muscular atrophy* (PSMA), a disease ultimately defined by finding only lower motor neuron pathology at autopsy, sparing the corticospinal tracts. Some authorities believe this syndrome may differ in etiology and pathogenesis from ALS because patients with PSMA tend to be younger and duration may be longer. But that has not been ascertained in sporadic ALS. In familial ALS, however, families with the A4V mutation in the gene for superoxide dismutase (SOD1) tend to have predominantly or solely lower motor neuron signs in life and the corticospinal tracts are often spared at autopsy.[3] In families with other mutations in the same gene, combinations of upper and motor neuron signs may differ in siblings or other first-degree relatives; there is not a strict correlation between the presence of any specific mutation and the appearance of upper motor neuron signs. The nature of this allelic heterogeneity is uncertain; it is not known whether other genes modify expression or environmental factors play a role.[4] Second, despite the lack of upper motor neuron signs in life, this patient could have had amyotrophic lateral sclerosis at autopsy, with degeneration in the corticospinal tracts as well as loss of motor neurons. There is no way to make that distinction in life, not if spinal muscular atrophy is defined strictly to include total loss of reflexes in a patient with weak, wasted, and visibly fasciculating muscles, with confirmatory evidence in the EMG. Combining data from previously published autopsy series,[5,6] only 7 of 23 patients with PSMA showed lesions restricted to the lower motor neurons. Sixteen patients showed degeneration of the pyramidal tracts although there had been no visible upper motor neuron signs in life. It is presumed that the overwhelming loss of the power motor neuron made it impossible for upper motor neuron signs to be expressed. In the most recent and largest autopsy series,[7] 23 of 120 cases had symptoms restricted to the lower motor neuron and 20 of the 23 showed corticospinal tract pathology. These patients did not differ in age at onset, duration of symptoms, or site of onset (bulbar or spinal) from those who had both upper and lower motor neuron signs in life. If this patient proved to have had ALS, he would have died of that disease without ever having been eligible to participate in a therapeutic trial because he did not meet criteria for 'definite' or 'probable' ALS.

Third, he could have had a motor neuropathy (MN). That is, he could have had a disorder of motor nerves without concomitant disease of sensory nerve fibers. This possibility is the crux of the diagnostic problem and it may be reasonably considered the most important problem in the differential diagnosis of ALS, because MN is a reversible disorder, lacking the lethal implications of ALS. In fact, this patient was first treated for a MN. A historical view of MN helps to explain the problem.

Rowland et al.[8] described a man who died after 2 years of a fasciculating lower motor neuron syndrome with slow motor nerve conduction and monoclonal gammopathy. The autopsy showed no loss of motor neurons but gave evidence of Wallerian degeneration. That patient was not studied specifically for conduction block, which had not yet become routine. Persistent conduction block was first described in 1982 by Lewis et al.,[9] who were studying patients with combined sensory and motor polyneuropathy, not strictly motor disorders. Then Chad, Parry and others[10-13] described patients with conduction block in purely motor neuropathies that clinically simulated motor neuron disease. In 1988, Pestronk et al.[14] described two patients with new features; both had antibodies to the neuronal ganglioside GM1 and both responded to cyclophosphamide therapy. In time it was found that the antibodies are present in fewer than half the cases, which is more prevalent than in ALS itself, but lack of antibodies does not exclude the diagnosis of MN. Then, IVIG therapy proved to be just as effective treatment, and safer.

One of the strange features of MN is the incongruous preservation of tendon reflexes in limbs with atrophic and fasciculating muscles; this pattern differs from the total absence of reflexes in PSMA and is one that had long been regarded as almost diagnostic of ALS. Yet conduction block is rarely found in patients with overt upper motor neuron signs.

Motor neuropathy is a peripheral neuropathy; it was first identified by and defined by the presence of conduction block and slow conduction. Demyelination of peripheral nerves (often the sensory sural nerve) has been found in biopsies; regenerative attempts may form masses or 'tomaculous' changes. One patient showed deposits of immunoglobulins at nodes of Ranvier.[15] Experimentally, gamma globulins from MN patients have blocked conduction in the peripheral nerve terminals of mice.[16]

Corbo et al.[17] found that numerous regenerative clusters were more characteristic of MN than ALS. The clusters in MN included Schwann cells but the clusters are small myelinated fibers, which are thought to form from two or more axonal sprouts that arise from proximal nerve fibers after the distal elements had undergone Wallerian degeneration. The sprouts grow together as a cluster within the residual basal lamina of the degenerated nerve fiber. In this case the clusters were present but not so numerous. These observed changes were partly the basis for the immunotherapy given to this patient.

Motor neuropathy includes some peculiar features. It is the only polyneuropathy that is purely motor in symptoms and signs. Also, with the possible exception of amyloid polyneuropathy, MN is the only polyneuropathy in which about half of reported cases show visible fasciculation, which is almost always a sign of disease of the perikaryon and MN is the only neuropathy in which half of all reported cases show active tendon jerks in limbs with weak, wasted and fasciculating muscles.

There has been debate about the relationship of MN to motor neuron disease. Peripheral neuropathy experts deride attempts to link the two. They state that no patient has ever improved if there were unequivocal upper motor neuron signs. Nevertheless, there have been only four published autopsies of patients with multifocal MN and conduction block.[18-21] Although all four showed changes in peripheral nerves or nerve roots, all four also showed loss of motor neurons. Two showed Bunina bodies in motor neurons and two showed changes in the corticospinal tracts. These are reliable histopathological signs of ALS. The patients also showed histopathological changes in peripheral or plexus nerves. Therefore, in a given case, both the perikaryon and the motor peripheral nerve may be affected; it does not have to be one or the other.[22]

Defining MN became more difficult in 1996, with reports that patients with the clinical syndrome might improve with IVIG therapy even if there were no conduction block, only slowing.[23,24] Then, Ellis et al.[25] found improvement even if there were no abnormalities at all in nerve conduction; their patients had a pure lower motor neuron syndrome. As in previous observations, the patients of Ellis et al. tended to be men; arms were affected more than legs; asymmetry was the rule; and, perhaps most important, the course was slow. The patient discussed here could have fallen into that category but did not respond to IVIG treatment.

Some authorities believe that MN is more closely related to chronic inflammatory demyelinating polyneuropathy (CIDP) than to motor neuron disease for several reasons: slow conduction velocity in both, implying demyelination; pathologic evidence of demyelination at sites of conduction block; and beneficial response to IVIG therapy. However, sensation is impaired clinically in CIDP, not in MN; this fact is not altered by reports of abnormal sensory conduction in MN. Active tendon reflexes and fasciculations are not seen in CIDP but are common in MN. The characteristically high CSF protein content and the beneficial effect of prednisone in CIDP are not evident in motor neuropathies. Slowing of motor conduction is more profound in CIDP, and relapses after improvement are more likely to occur in that condition. Abnormal titers of anti-GM1 are probably more common in MN. Authorities can take either side in this debate.

In practical terms, the diagnostic task is to differentiate between MN and the progressive spinal muscular atrophy form of ALS. That is now primarily the role of nerve conduction studies. However, new technologies are emerging. One is the use of motor nerve biopsies. Others include the use of magnetic resonance spectroscopy and magnetic stimulation of the motor cortex to identify disorders of the upper motor neuron. In the interim, it seems reasonable to try IVIG therapy in cases of solely lower motor neuron disorder or with retained tendon reflexes, especially those of long duration and slow progression.

One other aspect of this case is worth mentioning; namely, the monoclonal gammopathy. Although there has been no formal prospective case control study in a large population, Shy et al.[26] found that monoclonal paraproteinemia in 5% of ALS patients and only 1% of controls. That difference has been found in other studies as well. Also, some patients with gammopathy prove to have a lymphoproliferative disease. Whether the gammopathy here played any role in the pathogenesis is uncertain but there was no response to immunotherapy.[27]

Can we decide which of the three alternative diagnoses is correct? Against MN are the lack of physiological abnormalities of nerve conduction, the absence of anti-GM1 antibodies, the lack of response to IVIG, and a duration of symptoms less than 5 years. MN is also much less common than motor neuron disease.

Even if that consideration narrows the choices, the authors do not believe that, in this case, there can be a clinical choice between PSMA and ALS with predominantly lower motor neuron signs. The distinction has to be made at autopsy.

Clinical diagnosis

- Spinal muscular atrophy form of motor neuron disease, or
- amyotrophic lateral sclerosis, predominantly lower motor neuron form.
- Monoclonal gammopathy, IgG lambda, uncertain significance.

Post-mortem examination

The general autopsy showed no major concomitant disease. Specifically, there was no lymphoproliferative disease. CNS findings were as follows: Cortical sections showed spongiform changes in layers 1 and 2, most prominent in the precentral gyrus. Mild loss of Betz cells was accompanied by mild gliosis. Degeneration of the lateral and anterior descending corticospinal tracts was mild but was clear with luxol fast blue/para-amino salicylic acid (LFB/PAS) stains of the spinal cord. There were no collections of macrophages or loss of myelinated fibers in the internal capsule, cerebral peduncle, or pons. Neuronal loss was prominent in the hypoglossal nucleus. In the spinal cord there was loss of large motor neurons and mild gliosis. Remaining motor neurons were shrunken and Bunina bodies were rare, but present. An incidental finding was capillary telangiectasia in the pons and medulla.

Conclusions

This case demonstrates the importance of post-mortem examination, which is still the only way to ascertain the diagnosis of ALS. Evidence of both upper and lower motor neuron disease is the most common set of findings, even among cases like this one that are restricted to lower motor neuron signs in life. For reasons not clear, the perikaryal damage comes first and becomes so severe that upper motor neuron signs are never expressed. This is true regardless of whether the disease is sporadic or familial.

Some cases are restricted to the lower motor neuron and the corticospinal tracts are spared at autopsy. It is unclear whether that is another form of ALS or a distinct and different motor neuron disease.

The post-mortem findings in this case also illustrate the diagnostic value of finding Bunina bodies and hyaline inclusion bodies, which are now taken as reliable indicators of ALS.

Diagnosis

Amyotrophic lateral sclerosis, lower motor neuron dominant.

Clinical diagnosis: progressive spinal muscular atrophy with monoclonal gammopathy.

Anatomic diagnosis: amyotrophic lateral sclerosis.

References

1. Chan S, Shungu DC, Douglas-Akinwande AC, Lange DJ, Rowland LP. Motor neuron diseases: comparison of single-voxel, proton MR spectroscopy of the motor cortex with MR imaging of the brain in motor neuron diseases. *Radiology* 1999; **212**: 763–769.
2. World Federation of Neurology. El Escorial Criteria for the diagnosis of amyotrophic lateral sclerosis. *J Neurol Sci* 1994; **124** (suppl.): 96–107.
3. Cudkowicz ME, McKenna-Yasek R, Chen C et al. Limited corticospinal tract involvement in amyotrophic lateral sclerosis subjects with the A4V mutation in the copper/zinc superoxide dismutase gene. *Ann Neurol* 1998; **43**: 703–710.
4. Rowland LP. What's in a name? Amyotrophic lateral sclerosis, motor neuron disease, and allelic heterogeneity. *Ann Neurol* 1998; **43**: 691–694.
5. Brownell B, Oppenheimer DR, Hughes JT. Central nervous system in motor neuron disease. *J Neurol Neurosurg Psychiatry* 1970; **33**: 338–357.
6. Lawyer T Jr, Netsky MG. Amyotrophic lateral sclerosis: clinico-anatomic study of 53 cases. *Arch Neurol Psychiatry* 1953; **69**: 171–92.
7. Leung D, Kerikaya G, Hays AP, Rowland LP. Clinicopathological correlations in postmortem examination of 120 patients with motor neuron disease and analysis of neuronal inclusions in 40 patients. In preparation.
8. Rowland LP, Defendini R, Sherman W, Hirano A, Olarte MR, Latov N, Lovelace RE, Inoue K, Osserman EF. Macroglobulinemia with peripheral neuropathy simulating motor neuron disease. *Ann Neurol* 1982; **11**: 532–536.
9. Lewis RA, Sumner AJ, Brown MJ et al. Multifocal demyelinating neuropathy with persistent conduction block. *Neurology* 1982; **32**: 958–964.
10. Parry GJ, Clarke S. Multifocal acquired demyelinating neuropathy masquerading as motor neuron disease. *Muscle Nerve* 1988; **11**: 103–107.
11. Parry GJ, Holtz S, Hen-Zeev D, Drori JB. Gammopathy with proximal motor axonopathy simulating motor neuron disease. *Neurology* 1986; **36**: 273–276.
12. Roth G, Magistris MR. Neuropathies with conduction block, single and grouped fasciculations, localized limb myokymia. *EEG Clin Neurophysiol* 1987; **67**: 428–438.

13. Chad DA, Hammer K, Sargent J. Slow resolution of multifocal weakness and fasciculation: a reversible motor neuron syndrome. *Neurology* 1986; **36:** 1260–1263.
14. Pestronk A, Cornblath DR, Ilyas AA, Baba H, Quarles RH, Griffin JW, Alderson K, Adams RN. A treatable multifocal motor neuropathy with antibodies to GM1 ganglioside. *Ann Neurol* 1988; **24:** 73–78.
15. Santoro M, Thomas FP, Fink ME, Lange DJ, Uncini A, Wadia NH, Lator N, Hays AP. IgM deposits at nodes of Ranvier in a patient with amyotrophic lateral sclerosis, anti-GM1 antibodies, and multifocal motor conduction block. *Ann Neurol* 1990; **28:** 373–377.
16. Roberts M, Willison HJ, Paterson G, O'Hanlon G, Vincent A, Newsom-Davis J. Human monoclonal anti-GM1 ganglioside antibodies derived from multifocal motor neuropathy patients block distal motor nerve conduction. *Ann Neurol* 1995; **38:** 111–118.
17. Corbo M, Abouzahr MK, Latov N, Iannaccone S, Quattrini A, Nenni R, Canal N, Hays AP. Motor nerve biopsy studies in motor neuropathy and motor neuron disease. *Muscle Nerve* 1997; **20:** 15–21.
18. Adams D, Kuntzer T, Steck AJ, Lobrinus A, Janzer RC, Regli F. Motor conduction block and high titres of anti-GM1 ganglioside antibodies; pathological evidence of a motor neuropathy in a patient with lower motor neuron syndrome. *J Neurol Neurosurg Psychiatry* 1993; **56:** 982–987.
19. Oh SJ, Claussen GC, Odabasi Z, Palmer CP. Multifocal demyelinating motor neuropathy: pathologic evidence of 'inflammatory demyelinating polyradiculoneuropathy'. *Neurology* 1995; **45:** 1828–1832.
20. Veugelers B, Theys P, Lammends M, Van Hees J, Robberecht W. Pathological findings in a patient with amyotrophic lateral sclerosis and multifocal motor neuropathy with conduction block. *J Neurol Sci* 1996; **136:** 64–70.
21. Molinuevo JL, Cruz-Martinez A, Graus F, Serra J, Ribalta T, Vallis-Sole J. Central motor conduction time in patients with multifocal motor conduction block. *Muscle Nerve* 1999; **22:** 926–932.
22. Rowland LP. Muscular atrophies, motor neuropathies, amyotrophic lateral sclerosis and immunology. In: Kimura J, Kaji R, eds. *Physiology of ALS and Related Diseases*. Amsterdam: Elsevier Science, 1997: 3–11.
23. Pakiam A, Parry G. Multifocal motor neuropathy without evidence of conduction block. *Neurology* 1996; **46:** A234.
24. Katz JS, Wolfe GI, Bryan WW, Jackson CE, Amato AA, Barohn RJ. Electrophysiologic findings in multifocal motor neuropathy. *Neurology* 1997; **48:** 700–707.
25. Ellis CM, Leary S, Payan J, Shaw D, Hu M, O'Brien M, Leigh PN. Use of human intravenous immunoglobulin in lower motor neuron syndromes. *J Neurol Neurosurg Psychiatry* 1999; **67:** 15–19.
26. Shy ME, Rowland LP, Smith TS, Trojaborg W, Latov N, Sherman WH, Pesce MA, Lovelace RE, Osserman EF. Motor neuron disease and plasma cell dyscrasia. *Neurology* 1986; **36:** 1429–1436.
27. Rowland LP. Amyotrophic lateral sclerosis with paraproteins and autoantibodies. In: Serratrice G, Munsat T, eds. *Pathogenesis and Therapy of Amyotrophic Lateral Sclerosis*, vol. 68 (Advances in Neurology). Philadelphia: Lippincott-Raven, 1995: 93–105.

A case of fidgetiness and tics

Clinical history and examination

A 14-year-old boy was referred by his General Practitioner (GP) for evaluation of 'hyperactivity and involuntary movements.' His first symptom was noted at the age of 6 in the form of excessive eye blinking. Since then he has had a wide repertoire of movements such as flicking the head, nose twitch, facial grimace, shoulder shrug, arm and leg jerks, abdominal contractions and a torso twist. At the age of 11 years, he started to smell things and sniff, followed by grunting and making strange noises in his throat as if it needed constant clearing. Soon he began to repeat words and phrases he heard on TV, and would repeat his own sentence or the last word of a sentence. In addition he had an urge to imitate what other people did. He also started 'counting in his head' and felt forced to touch things. He was very meticulous with a concern for symmetry and to do things 'just right.' He also had some 'rituals' such as folding things in a particular way and turning knobs on doors a certain number of times. Other behaviors included hitting himself and banging his head on the wall.

His birth and early development were reported to be normal. However, his mother reported that he was 'always on the go as if driven by a motor'; he was restless and fidgety, climbing onto things, excitable and impulsive, had no sense of danger and seemed to act without thinking. At junior school, teachers often complained that he was hyperactive and distractible, and was unable to concentrate in class and often looked as if he was not listening.

His symptoms waxed and waned and he could suppress them voluntarily for brief periods of time, though this increased inner tension. When this tension mounted up too much there seemed to be a rebound increase in his symptoms. The type and nature of movements would also change at times, with old ones disappearing and new ones developing. The symptoms were made worse by tiredness and stress while it was better when he was relaxing, or concentrating on something. When he was 14 years of age, he started to say 'fu, fu' and then one day he said the full 'F word' followed by a cough as if to cover it up and he became extremely upset at this. Any type of swearing was out of character for him. An urgent appointment was made with the GP who then referred him to a pediatrician. He was started on methylphenidate (Ritalin) which improved his concentration and hyperactivity but his movements worsened. A further referral was hence made to a movement disorder clinic.

Neurological and mental state examination were normal apart from the motor and vocal tics. Investigations including full blood count, acanthocytes, urea and electrolytes, thyroid and liver function tests, serum copper, ceruloplasmin, uric acid, EEG, and CT scan were all within normal limits. Neuropsychological assessment and IQ as well as chromosomal analysis were normal.

On careful evaluation, it was found that his mother had checking behaviors (gas, doors, lights) and a maternal uncle had a nose and facial twitch as well as throat clearing.

*   *   *

Discussion

The patient was started on clonidine with good response and this was maintained 2 years later with no side-effects. Prior to starting on clonidine an ECG was performed (normal) and his blood pressure was measured (normal).

Gilles de la Tourettes syndrome (TS) is characterized by both multiple motor and one or more vocal tics which last for longer than a year and begin in childhood or early adolescence.[1,2] The generally accepted prevalence for TS used to be around 0.42–0.5 per 1000 (i.e. 4.28–5 per 10 000),[3,4] although other studies have yielded higher rates. More recently it has been demonstrated that it is much more common than previously suggested with a prevalence rate of 2.9% in mainstream secondary school children.[5] In children with special educational needs and learning disabilities, rates of 26%[6] and 24%,[7] respectively have been observed. Tourettes syndrome is found in all cultures, countries and racial groups and occurs three to four times more commonly in males.[8,9]

Clinical characteristics

Tourettes syndrome patients share a similar clinical profile irrespective of culture, underlying the biological nature of the condition. In the majority of studies it has been noted that TS starts at the age of 5–7 with motor tics (such as excessive eye blinking), followed by the vocal tics around the age of 11 (such as throat clearing and sniffing). Coprolalia (the involuntary and inappropriate uttering of obscenities), when present, usually begins at a later age of around 15 years.[9] It has also been suggested that the majority of symptoms disappear in about half of the patients by the age of 18 years.[10] Commonly reported motor tics are eye blinking, facial grimacing, nose twitching, mouth opening, head nodding, neck stretching and shoulder shrugging and the most common vocal tics are sniffing, throat clearing, snorting, gulping, squeaking, and yelping. Complex motor tics are common in TS and include touching, licking, spitting, jumping, smelling, squatting, twirling and abnormalities of gait.

It may be clinically useful to subdivide TS into three types.[11] (i) The first is simple TS (with motor and vocal tics being the predominant and almost only symptoms). (ii) Second is 'full blown TS' (with coprolalia – inappropriate uttering of obscenities; copropraxia – the inappropriate making of obscene gestures; echolalia – copying what other people say; echopraxia – copying other peoples' movements; palilalia – repeating the end of one's own sentence; and palipraxia – repeating one's own behaviors). (iii) Thirdly, there may be 'TS plus' (originally described by Packer[12]) in which the TS patients may also have attention deficit hyperactivity disorder (ADHD); obsessive–compulsive behaviors (OCB); self-injurious behaviors (SIB), and other psychopathology.

Secondary Tourettism[13] as well as tics and TS symptoms starting for the first time in late adult life have been reported. It has been suggested that adult onset tic disorders consist of idiopathic and secondary tics, and in comparison with DSM classified younger onset cases, they may have more severe symptoms, presence of a potential trigger event, increased sensitivity and poor response to neuroleptic medication and a lower frequency of spontaneous remission.[14,15] Several cases of secondary Tourettism has been described in the literature and the causes include post-encephalic syndrome, carbon monoxide intoxication, degenerative and vascular etiologies, trauma, infections, alcohol withdrawal, exposure to drugs such as amphetamines, neuroleptics and anticholinergics. It has also been observed that an environmental event may unmask the symptoms in later life in a constitutionally predisposed individual.

Recent research has suggested that tics and associated behaviors including OCB might develop from streptococcal infection by the process of molecular mimicry, whereby antibodies directed against bacterial antigens cross-react with brain targets. It is postulated that this may have a direct etiological role or may act to modulate the phenotypic expression of TS, and in this regard anti-neuronal antibodies have been demonstrated in association with involuntary repetitive movement disorders. This spectrum of neurobehavioral disorders have been termed pediatric autoimmune neuropsychiatric disorders associated with streptococcal infection (PANDAS).[16,17] Although interesting and novel, however, the notion is still a matter of controversy and the use of immune modifying therapies in these situations also need further controlled studies.[18,19]

In TS patients, regional cerebral blood flow studies using positron emission tomography (PET) and single photon emission tomography (SPET) have reported abnormalities in the basal ganglia and frontal cortex.[20] Magnetic resonance imaging (MRI) has shown left/right asymmetries in the basal ganglia and reduction in basal ganglia volumes in TS.[21] Furthermore, dopamine D2-receptor availability studies have shown lower binding of the ^{123}I-IBZM in the basal ganglia of TS patients.[22]

Investigations and differential diagnosis

Investigations are mainly carried out to rule out other movement disorders and these include Sydenhams chorea, Huntingtons disease, acanthocytosis, tardive Tourettism in response to neuroleptic medication, spasmodic torticollis, Wilsons disease and myoclonic epilepsy. There are no specific EEG changes in TS. Neurophysiological and neuropsychological assessments have also not revealed any specific abnormalities. In patients with self-injurious behaviors, it is important to rule out Leisch–Nyhan syndrome.

Treatment

Chemotherapy is the mainstay of treatment for the motor and vocal tics and traditionally includes dopamine blockers such as haloperidol, pimozide, sulpiride, tiapride and risperidone. The doses of neuroleptics given in TS are low (e.g. haloperidol 1.5 mg daily) in contrast to the functional psychosis, where substantially larger doses may be given. Treatment of TS and ADHD pose a major therapeutic challenge, as stimulants such as methyl phenidate, although effective for ADHD, may worsen the tics. In these situations, clonidine may well be the treatment of choice as it is known to improve both tics and ADHD. Specific serotonin re-uptake inhibitors (SSRIs) have been successfully used to treat OCB symptoms and in such instances these agents are used in combination with dopamine blockers. Other neuroleptics (such as fluphenazine, and penfluridol) the anticonvulsant clonazepam, calcium antagonists like nifedipine and verapamil, naloxone, nicotine, lithium carbonate, tetrabenazine, progabide, marijuana, metoclopramide, cholinergic agents such as physostigmine, muscarinic compounds like RS-86, dopamine agonist like pergolide, androgen receptor blocker such as flutamide, and local injection of botulinum toxin, etc. have all been used with reports of some success.[23,24]

In addition to pharmacotherapy, psychosocial interventions form an important component of TS management. Both the TS individual and the family often benefit from support groups. In a few patients, symptom exacerbation may occur in relation to allergy or certain food items, and these patients may benefit from appropriate interventions.

Diagnosis

Gilles de la Tourrettes syndrome with attention deficit hyperactivity disorder (ADHD).

References

1. American Psychiatric Association. *Diagnostic and Statistical Manual of Mental Disorders (Fourth edition) (DSM-IV)*. Washington, DC: American Psychiatric Association, 1994.
2. World Health Organization. *International Classification of Diseases and Health Related Problems*, Tenth Revision. Geneva: World Health Organization, 1992.
3. Apter A, Pauls DL, Bleich et al. An epidemiologic study of Gilles de la Tourette's syndrome in Israel. *Arch Gen Psychiatry* 1993; **50:** 734–738.
4. Bruun, RD. Gilles de la Tourette's syndrome: an overview of clinical experience. *J Am Acad Child Adolesc Psychiatry* 1984, **23:** 126–133.
5. Mason A, Banerjee S, Eapen V et al. The prevalence of Tourette syndrome in a mainstream school population. *Dev Med Child Neurol* 1998; **40:** 292–296.
6. Kurlan R, Whitmore D, Irvine C et al. Tourette's syndrome in a special education population: a pilot study involving a single school district. *Neurology* 1994; **44:** 699–702.
7. Eapen V, Robertson MM, Zeitlin H et al. Gilles de la Tourette's syndrome in special education schools: a United Kingdom study. *J Neurol* 1997; **244:** 378–382.
8. Robertson MM. The Gilles de la Tourette syndrome: the current status. *Br J Psychiatry* 1989; **154:** 147–169.
9. Robertson MM. Annotation: Gilles de la Tourette syndrome – an update. *J Child Psychol Psychiatry* 1994; **35:** 597–611.
10. Leckman JF, Zhang H, Vitale A et al. Course of tic severity in Tourette syndrome: the first two decades. *Pediatrics* 1998; **102:** 14–19.
11. Robertson MM, Baron-Cohen S. *Tourette Syndrome: The Facts.* Oxford: Oxford University Press, 1998.
12. Packer LE. Social and educational resources for patients with Tourette syndrome. *Neurol Clin* 1997; **15:** 457–473.
13. Jankovic J. Diagnosis and classification of tics and Tourette syndrome. *Adv Neurol* 1992; **58:** 7–14.
14. Chouinard S, Fahn S, Ford B. Adult onset tic disorders. *Neurology* 1997; **48:** A398.
15. Eapen V., Lees AJ, Lakke JPWF et al. Adult onset Gilles de la Tourette syndrome. *Mov Disord*, in press.
16. Swedo SE, Leonard HL, Mittleman, BB et al. Identification of children with pediatric autoimmune neuropsychiatric disorders associated with streptococcal infections by a marker associated with rheumatic fever. *Am J Psychiatry* 1997; **154:** 110–112.

17. Swedo SE, Leonard HL, Garvey M et al. Pediatric autoimmune neuropsychiatric disorders associated with streptococcal infections: clinical description of the first 50 cases. *Am J Psychiatry* 1998; **155:** 264–271.
18. Kurlan R. Investigating Tourette syndrome as a neurologic sequela of rheumatic fever. *CNS Spectrums* 1999; **4:** 62–67.
19. Kurlan R. Tourette's syndrome and 'PANDAS': will the relation bear our? Pediatric autoimmune neuropsychiatric disorders associated with streptococcal infection. *Neurology* 1998; **50:** 1618–1624.
20. Moriarty J, Eapen V, Costa DC et al. HMPAO SPECT does not distinguish obsessive compulsive and tic syndromes in families multiply affected with Gilles de la Tourette syndrome. *Psychol Med* 1997; **27:** 737–740.
21. Greco A. Structural neuroimaging: magnetic resonance. In: Robertson MM, Eapen V, eds. *Movement and Allied Disorders in Childhood.* New York: John Wiley, 1995: 279–292.
22. Alexander GE. Functional neuroanatomy of basal ganglia. In: Robertson MM, Eapen V, eds. *Movement and Allied Disorders in Childhood.* New York: John Wiley, 1995: 257–278.
23. Eapen V, Robertson MM. Gilles de la Tourette syndrome and co-morbid obsessive compulsive disorder. Therapeutic interventions. *CNS Drugs* 2000; **13:** 173–183.
24. Robertson MM. Invited review. Tourette Syndrome, associated conditions and the complexities of treatment. *Brain* 2000; **123:** 425–462.

Paresthesias and a cerebral mass

The patient was a 43-year-old, right-handed woman who presented in 1991 with a 1-year history of intermittent paresthesias in both hands. This was not accompanied by numbness or weakness and the paresthesias intensified over the 6 weeks prior to her admission. In the month prior to admission, she began to experience paresthesias of the right leg and a sensation of heaviness in both legs. She had trouble keeping up with her young children and had a tendency to drag the right leg. She also developed paresthesias in the perineal region without any disturbance of bowel or bladder function. The patient thought her memory was unaffected, but she acknowledged that she did not feel mentally clear. She had no headaches, visual or bulbar symptoms and no back pain.

The patient did not smoke or drink alcohol. There had been no recent travel. She had no prior neurologic symptoms or medical illnesses. There was no history of hypertension, diabetes, or any chronic illness. She did not take any medications. There was no family history of neurologic disease.

On examination her blood pressure was 110/70. She was afebrile. Her pulse was 90 and regular. The patient looked healthy and fit and was in no distress. Her general medical examination was entirely normal including rectal tone and anal wink. On neurologic exam, mental status and cranial nerves were normal. Motor testing revealed a mild right hemiparesis as evidenced by slowed rapid alternating movements in the right hand, as well as mild weakness of wrist extension and intrinsic muscles of the right hand. She had mild weakness of flexion and extension of the right foot and the hamstring muscles on the right. All primary sensory modalities were intact to formal testing, although the patient did have an ill-defined allodynia in the right leg. Stereognosis was normal. Her gait was normal

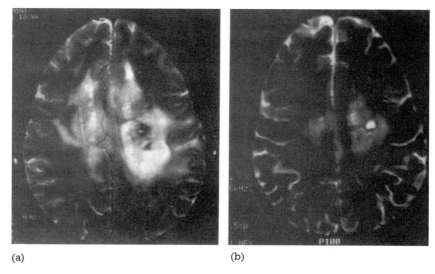

(a)   (b)

Fig. 8.1. T2-weighted MR images demonstrating an extensive, infiltrative, bilateral tumor (a). The lesion has substantially diminished in size after chemotherapy (b).

save for reduced arm swing on the right and inability to walk on her heels with her right foot. Reflexes were notable for being diffusely brisk throughout the right arm and leg but no Babinski was evident.

Complete blood count, electrolytes, hepatic and renal function tests were normal. A cranial MR scan was performed which revealed an extensive non-enhancing mass primarily confined to the white matter (Fig. 8.1). The lesion predominantly involved the left centrum semiovale but crossed the corpus callosum and involved the right side as well. In November 1992, the patient underwent a stereotactic needle biopsy.

*   *   *

Discussion

The biopsy revealed a low-grade oligodendroglioma. Post-operatively, the patient was maintained on dexamethasone for several weeks. Prior to the start of treatment the patient became irrational and developed an acute confusional state characterized by paranoia, irritability and perseveration. On examination, she had normal memory and cognitive function but clearly exhibited paranoid ideation. The patient was hospitalized and a repeat cranial MRI was unchanged. Cerebrospinal fluid was normal as well as CBC, electrolytes and liver function tests. Electroencephalogram did not reveal any epileptiform activity. Her symptoms were attributed to a steroid-induced psychosis. She was treated with haloperidol and her dexamethasone was tapered and discontinued. She made a full recovery and has had no recurrence of similar symptoms since.

Many patients with low-grade gliomas can be followed initially, but this patient's mild but progressive hemiparesis and subtle cognitive dysfunction necessitated treatment of the tumor. She was started on combination chemotherapy using procarbazine, lomustine (CCNU) and vincristine (PCV). She completed seven cycles of PCV by the end of 1993. Her chemotherapy course was complicated by the development of a hypersensitivity rash to procarbazine after the second cycle and it was deleted from further cycles of chemotherapy. After the third cycle, vincristine was discontinued because of peripheral neuropathy; consequently, the last four cycles of chemotherapy consisted of CCNU alone. She developed only mild to moderate myelosuppression throughout the course of treatment. She had no infectious or bleeding complications during therapy nor did she require any transfusions.

The patient followed with serial MR scans during her treatment. She had a definite but incomplete shrinkage of her non-enhancing lesion which has been stable since (Fig. 8.1). She also experienced a clinical improvement with resolution of her right-sided weakness and return of her mental function to normal. She was last seen in 2000 and had a stable MR scan and stable neurologic function.

This patient presented with progressive symptoms and signs of a mild right hemiparesis and cognitive impairment which were primarily subjective. Her neuroimaging was markedly abnormal and explained her neurologic condition. The MRI shows a diffuse, non-enhancing abnormality primarily confined to the hemispheric white matter. The lesion is bilateral, infiltrates the corpus callosum, and is confluent. It occupies space as evidenced by compression of the lateral ventricles. It involves a much larger area of brain than anticipated on the basis of her neurologic symptoms and signs. In fact, she is relatively intact compared with the extensive abnormality seen on MRI. The history of subacute, progressive neurologic dysfunction, combined with this diffuse non-enhancing space-occupying abnormality on neuroimaging, is consistent with only one diagnosis – an infiltrating brain tumor. The lesions are too large and confluent to represent cerebrovascular disease in this relatively young woman without any risk factors. Furthermore, her clinical syndrome did not suggest a stroke as there was no acute event and her symptoms evolved over many months. Although the non-enhancing abnormality is periventricular, the lesion is too confluent to represent multiple sclerosis. She has no history of relapsing or remitting neurologic symptoms and has relatively few signs for such extensive disease due to demyelination. These diagnoses seem very unlikely.

Primary brain tumors typically infiltrate widely in the brain and, in particular, track through the white matter. Primary central nervous system lymphomas (PCNSL) are characteristically periventricular in location but almost always have some enhancement, particularly in immunocompetent individuals.[1] The absence of enhancement, and the diffuse confluent bilateral nature of the lesion, makes PCNSL unlikely. Furthermore, PCNSL remains an uncommon disease even though it has increased in incidence across the USA.

Gliomas are highly infiltrative tumors that can involve large regions of brain without producing many clinical symptoms or signs.[2,3] They primarily involve hemispheric white matter, and tumor cells can migrate extensively without destroying the underlying brain tissue. This accounts for the relative paucity of neurologic deficits in this patient, despite such widespread involvement of brain.

Gliomas are easily identified by MR scans. In this patient, the absence of contrast enhancement strongly suggests the tumor is low grade, whereas contrast enhancement typically characterizes a high-grade glioma.[4] Contrast enhancement is indicative of disruption of the blood–brain barrier which parallels the development of neovascularity, one of the pathologic hallmarks of malignant gliomas. In low grade lesions, the lack of contrast enhancement suggests the majority of tumor resides behind a relatively intact blood–brain barrier despite extensive involvement of brain. This patient has a diffuse tumor which involves both hemispheres, but all the disease is protected by the blood–brain barrier. Gliomas are the most common primary brain tumors and astrocytomas are more common than oligodendrogliomas. In the past, the distinction between astrocytic and oligodendroglial neoplasms was of little therapeutic importance. Consequently, pathologists often did not focus on subtle distinctions between these two types of neoplasms or note the presence of dual pathologic features in a single tumor, the so-called 'mixed glioma.' With the increasing recognition that oligodendrogliomas are uniquely chemosensitive, the incidence of diagnosis of oligodendrogliomas is rising.[5,6] Whether this represents an appreciation of the true incidence of these unusual neoplasms, or the pathologist's eagerness to identify even a small area of oligodendroglial cells within a predominantly astrocytic neoplasm which confers a better prognosis, is unclear.

Neuroradiologically, it is impossible to distinguish an astrocytic from an oligodendroglial neoplasm with any certainty. Oligodendroglial tumors frequently calcify, and even low-grade tumors may be associated with a propensity for intracranial hemorrhage. However, these are not absolutes, and even low-grade astrocytic lesions can have calcifications, or rarely, hemorrhage. Therefore, histologic examination is essential to make a specific diagnosis. However, there is considerable controversy on the importance of making an immediate diagnosis of a low-grade glioma in a patient with a typical clinical syndrome and radiographic image. This is particularly true for patients, such as this patient, in whom surgical resection is impossible.

Although controversial, most neuro-oncologists believe that complete resection of a tumor, even a low-grade brain tumor, prolongs survival.[7,8] When a lesion typical of a low-grade glioma is located in an area such as the frontal pole or temporal tip, which is amenable to complete resection, most tumor specialists would advocate extirpation of the lesion. This would allow for complete histologic evaluation and tumor typing and would also serve as an initial therapy. Complete resection rarely results in cure since most tumors are associated with malignant cells that have infiltrated brain at a distance from the area of bulk disease but these areas cannot be appreciated as abnormal on current neuroimaging techniques. Consequently, the resection of all identifiable disease usually leaves behind microscopic tumor that eventually regrows in the future. Nevertheless, complete resection of low-grade lesions has been associated with prolonged survival. However, most low-grade tumors are not amenable to extirpation. Many involve the insular cortex or infiltrate critical regions of brain, preventing surgical removal. Biopsy, often stereotactic biopsy, is the only method to obtain tissue for diagnosis.

Biopsy can provide tissue for diagnosis, but gliomas are frequently very heterogeneous tumors. They may be low grade throughout, but have features of astrocytoma or oligodendroglioma in different regions. Biopsy will only reflect the pathology of the area sampled and may mislead the treating physician as to the predominant histology of the tumor as a whole. In addition, most low-grade tumors transform into high grade malignancies. Often, this transformation occurs within a focal location of an otherwise low-grade glioma.[9] Occasionally, but not always, focal transformation is evident radiographically by small areas of enhancement within a non-enhancing lesion.[10] When this is seen, the biopsy should be targeted to the enhancement, since treatment is defined by the most malignant component of the tumor. In completely non-enhancing tumors, identification of malignant foci can sometimes be accomplished by positron emission tomography (PET) scan, enabling the neurosurgeon to direct his biopsy to areas of hypermetabolism which correlates with anaplasia.[11,12] At the Memorial Sloan-Kettering Cancer Center, we perform a PET scan on all patients with presumed low-grade gliomas to guide biopsy or subsequent therapy.

In patients who first present with what appears to be a low-grade glioma, how important is it to make a histologic diagnosis immediately?[13] Most low-grade gliomas, particularly those in young adults, present with seizures in a patient who is otherwise neurologically intact. The majority of these patients can have their seizures controlled with anticonvulsants and do not require immediate treatment of their tumor to achieve symptom control.[13,14] The cornerstone of treatment for low-grade gliomas has been radiotherapy. However, at present it is unclear whether administering radiotherapy at diagnosis either improves survival or neurologic outcome as opposed to deferring treatment until it is symptomatically required. Two randomized prospective trials demonstrated that low dose immediate radiotherapy (45–50.4 Gy) was as effective as higher doses (59.4–64.8 Gy), but those receiving higher doses had worse levels of functioning and a greater symptom burden.[15,16] The European Organization for Research and Treatment of Cancer (EORTC) also completed a randomized trial of histologically confirmed low-grade gliomas.[17] They randomized patients to immediate versus deferred radiotherapy (54 Gy) until patients developed clinically or radiographically progressive tumor. These data are the first to address definitely the issue of whether early radiation benefits patients. Patients who had deferred radiation had a reduced progression-free survival (37%) at 5 years compared with those who had immediate radiation (44%, $P = 0.02$), but overall survival was identical in the two groups. Furthermore, patients who underwent immediate radiation had a higher incidence of radiation-related toxicity. Consequently, survival is not compromised by deferring radiation until patients develop symptoms that mandate treatment, and they experience less toxicity.

While most patients with low-grade gliomas present with seizures, a minority will present with cognitive impairment or progressive lateralizing symptoms and signs. Immediate treatment is often essential in such patients to control neurologic symptoms and to prevent, or at least delay, further progression. In such patients, there is no consideration of deferring treatment. These patients include those whose seizures cannot be controlled with anticonvulsants. In such patients, biopsy or resection should be performed immediately and appropriate treatment instituted. In patients with classic radiographic low-grade gliomas who have seizures easily controlled with anticonvulsants, and in whom treatment would not be instituted immediately even if the histologic diagnosis is established, one can safely defer biopsy until the time of tumor progression. A retrospective study done by Recht et al.[13] has demonstrated the safety of this approach which has also been confirmed in subsequent studies.[14,18]

This patient had progressive lateralizing symptoms and signs which would necessitate treatment of a histologically confirmed low-grade glioma. Consequently, she underwent immediate biopsy and pathology established this was a low-grade oligodendroglioma. Treatment of low-grade astrocytomas consists of involved field radiotherapy; however, treatment of low-grade oligodendrogliomas is controversial and optimal initial treatment has not been established. Low-grade oligodendrogliomas can be effectively treated with radiotherapy and, historically, this has been the standard approach. However, concern about the long-term cognitive consequences of radiotherapy, particularly when lesions are large and bilateral as in this patient, and the recognition that such tumors may be chemosensitive, have prompted many neuro-oncologists to initiate treatment of even low-grade oligodendrogliomas with chemotherapy.

The chemosensitivity of oligodendroglial tumors has primarily been established in the much rarer malignant oligodendroglioma.[19] In the malignant oligodendroglioma, 75% of patients will respond to the combination chemotherapy regimen of PCV. Chemosensitivity of low-grade oligodendrogliomas is less clear and a large study has not been performed.[20,21] However, there is anecdotal evidence to suggest that low-grade tumors can respond well to chemotherapy and that low-grade mixed gliomas have an intermediate responsiveness between the pure oligodendroglioma and the pure astrocytoma.

In malignant oligodendrogliomas, chemosensitivity has been linked to specific cytogenetic abnormalities, specifically loss of chromosome 1p.[22] Loss of heterozygosity (LOH) of 1p correlates very highly with chemosensitivity, whereas the absence of 1p LOH predicts chemoresistance. This relationship seems quite tight for malignant oligodendrogliomas and has recently been examined in low-grade oligodendrogliomas where preliminary data also link chemosensitivity to 1p LOH.[23] These data have yet to be confirmed and, therefore, molecular analysis of low grade oligodendrogliomas should not necessarily be used to guide specific treatment decisions.

This patient has had a substantial and durable response to treatment that has now lasted for more than 9 years. She has had a complete clinical resolution of her symptoms and signs, although substantial abnormality remains on neuroimaging. This exemplifies one of the hallmarks of low-grade glial neoplasms. Because they infiltrate widely but do not destroy underlying brain tissue, effective treatment of the tumor can often result in substantial clinical improvement with no permanent deficits.

Large malignant glial tumors are characterized by a focal contrast enhancing mass. One of the pathologic features is neovascularity which is associated with an absence of the normal blood–brain barrier throughout the tumor. This allows for enhanced permeability with potentially improved access of systemically administered drug to tumor. Low-grade tumors are characterized by the absence of vascular changes. Individual cells can be seen infiltrating diffusely throughout the brain without disrupting the normal blood–brain barrier. This means that any systemic chemotherapeutic agent that is administered must penetrate a relatively intact blood–brain barrier to effectively treat the tumor. The PCV combination was designed, in part, to deliver drugs behind an intact blood–brain barrier. The procarbazine and CCNU are lipophilic and can penetrate the barrier to reach disease anywhere in the brain. Vincristine is incapable of penetrating the blood–brain barrier and its importance in the treatment of such a low-grade tumor is unclear. Oligodendrogliomas are primarily sensitive to alkylating agents such as procarbazine and CCNU.[24] Other agents reported to be effective in the treatment of this disease include melphalan and thiotepa. Drugs with other mechanisms of action, such as the platins and paclitaxel, may also be effective and have primarily been used at relapse.

It is unknown if chemotherapy is more or equally effective than radiotherapy for the treatment of oligodendrogliomas. Chemotherapy is frequently selected as the initial treatment as a means of deferring radiotherapy. Although radiotherapy is easy to administer and most patients suffer no acute toxicities, many long-term survivors do suffer memory and cognitive deficits as a consequence of cranial radiotherapy. This is an important issue, because long-term survival is common with oligodendrogliomas. A recent review of their experience at the Memorial Sloan-Kettering Cancer Center revealed a median survival of 16 years for low-grade oligodendrogliomas.[18] The review was retrospective, but failed to identify any difference in outcome using initial treatment with radiotherapy, chemotherapy or both. In addition, a large tumor which involves an extensive area of brain demands a large radiotherapy port, often encompassing the whole brain, which enhances the potential for late cognitive deficits. Once these deficits develop, they are irreversible; they may be static or progressive even in the absence of further treatment. This is the primary reason that chemotherapy is often selected over radiation as the initial treatment. Toxicities of chemotherapy are acute and usually related to myelosuppression; however, once treatment stops, the patient recovers and there is no known delayed effect upon the brain. There is a remote possibility that chemotherapy can lead to a second malignancy (particularly leukemia) in the future, but the risk is small. Ultimately, only long follow-up of such patients will help define the best approach to treatment of a newly diagnosed low grade oligodendroglioma.

Diagnosis

Low grade oligodendroglioma.

References

1. Raizer JJ, DeAngelis LM. Primary central nervous system lymphoma. In: Raghavan D, Brecher ML, Johnson DH, Meropol NJ, Moots PL, Thigpen JT, eds. *Textbook of Uncommon Cancer*, 2nd edn. New York: John Wiley, 1999: 323–333.
2. Mikkelsen T, Rosenblum ML. Tumor invasiveness. In: Berger MS, Wilson CB, eds. *The Gliomas*. WB Saunders, Philadelphia, 1999: 76–86.
3. Rogers LR, Weinstein MA, Estes ML et al. Diffuse bilateral cerebral astrocytomas with atypical neuroimaging studies. *J Neurosurg* 1994; **81:** 817–821.
4. Gold RL, Dillon WP Jr 1999. Magnetic Resonance Imaging. In: Berger MS, Wilson CB, eds. *The Gliomas*. WB Saunders, Philadelphia, 1999: 275–293.
5. Coons SW, Johnson PC, Scheithauer BW. Improving diagnostic accuracy and interobserver concordance in the classification and grading of primary gliomas. *Cancer* 1997; **79:** 1381–1393.
6. Fortin D, Cairncross GJ, Hammond RR. Oligodendroglioma: an appraisal of recent data pertaining to diagnosis and treatment. *Neurosurgery* 1999; **45:** 1279–1291.
7. Bampoe J, Bernstein M. The role of surgery in low-grade gliomas. *J Neuro-Oncol* 1999; **42:** 259–269.
8. Van Veelen ML, Avezaat CJ, Kros JM. Supratentorial low-grade astrocytoma: prognostic factors, dedifferentiation, and the issue of early versus late surgery. *J Neurol Neurosurg Psychiatry* 1998; **64:** 581–587.
9. Scully RE, Mark EJ, McNeely WF et al. Case records of the Massachusetts General Hospital. Case 12 – 1997. *New Engl J Med* 1997; **336:** 1163–1171.

10. Barker FG, Chang SM, Huhn SL et al. Age and the risk of anaplasia in magnetic resonance – nonenhancing supratentorial cerebral tumors. *Cancer* 1997; **80:** 936–941.

11. Thiel A, Pietrzyk U, Sturm V et al. Enhanced accuracy in differential diagnosis of radiation necrosis by positron emission tomography-magnetic resonance imaging coregistration: technical case report. *Neurosurgery* 2000; **46:** 232–234.

12. Goldman S, Levivier M, Pirotte B et al. Regional glucose metabolism and histopathology of gliomas. A study based on positron emission tomography-guided stereotactic biopsy. *Cancer* 1996; **78:** 1098–1106.

13. Recht LD, Lew R, Smith TW et al. Suspected low-grade glioma: is deferring treatment safe? *Ann Neurol* 1992; **31:** 431–436.

14. Bauman G, Lote K, Larson D et al. Pretreatment factors predict overall survival for patients with low-grade glioma: a recursive partitioning analysis. *Int J Radiat Oncol Biol Phys* 1999; **45:** 923–929.

15. Karim ABM, Maat B, Hatlevoll R et al. A randomized trial on dose–response in radiation therapy of low-grade cerebral gliomas. European Organization for Research and Treatment of Cancer (EORTC) Study 22844. *Int J Radiat Oncol Biol Phys* 1996; **36:** 549–556.

16. Shaw EG, Arussell R, Scheithauer BW et al. A prospective randomized trial of low- versus high-dose radiation therapy in adults with supratentorial low-grade glioma: initial report of a NCCTG–RTOG–ECOG study. *Proc Am Soc Clin Oncology* 1998; **17:** 401a.

17. Karim AB, Cornu P, Bleehen N et al. Immediate postoperative radiotherapy in low-grade glioma improves progression free survival, but not overall survival: preliminary results of an EORTC/MRC randomized phase III study. *Proc Am Soc Clin Oncol* 1998; **17:** 400a.

18. Olson JD, Riedel E, DeAngelis LM. Long-term outcome of low-grade oligodendroglioma and mixed glioma. *Neurology* 2000; **54:** 1442–1448.

19. Cairncross G, Macdonald D, Ludwin S et al. Chemotherapy for anaplastic oligodendroglioma. *J Clin Oncol* 1994; **12:** 2013–2021.

20. Mason WP, Krol SG, DeAngelis LM. Low-grade oligodendroglioma responds to chemotherapy. *Neurology* 1996; **46:** 203–207.

21. Glass J, Hochberg GH, Gruber ML et al. The treatment of oligodendrogliomas and mixed oligodendroglioma–astrocytomas with PCV chemotherapy. *J Neurosurg* 1992; **76:** 741–745.

22. Cairncross JG, Ueki K, Zlatescu MC et al. Specific genetic predictors of chemotherapeutic response and survival in patients with anaplastic oligodendrogliomas. *J Natl Cancer Inst* 1998; **90:** 1473–1479.

23. Smith JS, Perry A, Borell TJ et al. Alterations of chromosome arms 1p and 19q as predictors of survival in oligodendrogliomas, astrocytomas, and mixed oligoastrocytomas. *J Clin Oncol* 2000; **18:** 636–645.

24. Perry JR, Louis DN, Cairncross JG. Current treatment of oligodendrogliomas. *Arch Neurol* 1999; **56:** 434–436.

A frontal lobe mass lesion

Clinical history and examination

The patient was a 24-year-old woman who had frequent common migraine since age 17. She underwent neurologic examination at age 23 in December 1998. The findings were normal, as were cranial computed tomography (CT).

In late June 1999, at age 24, she noted difficulty walking. Her right leg felt clumsy. Within 1 week her right arm was weak. An episode of vertigo and nausea caused her to fall to the floor with brief loss of consciousness. Following that, the right-sided weakness worsened.

She was admitted to hospital 10 days after the onset. She was afebrile, pulse was 84, and blood pressure 100/70. She was alert, oriented, and had a normal mental status examination. General physical examination was normal. She had spastic weakness of the right arm, flaccid severe weakness of the right leg, and a Babinski sign on the right. She had no facial weakness. She could walk only a short distance with assistance because of the right leg weakness. Findings were otherwise normal.

On admission, WBC was 15.3, Hgb 11.4, hematocrit 35.2, and platelet count 235 000. Total protein was 6.7, albumin 3.6, calcium 8.8, magnesium 2.0, sodium 135, potassium 3.5, chloride 96, CO_2 27, BUN 16, creatinine 0.7. B12 level was 249, folate 15.8, PT was 10.5, INR 0.93, PTT 28.3, WSR 57. ANA was negative, and SSA and SSB antibody titers were negative.

Cerebrospinal fluid showed 0 WBC, protein of 23 mg %, glucose 60 mg %, oligoclonal bands were absent, and IgG synthesis rate was normal (2.1 mg/24 h). IgG concentration was 3.0 mg %, IgG index was 0.59, RPR was negative, and CSF Lyme titer was negative. Visual evoked potentials and auditory evoked potentials were normal.

Cranial MRI (Fig. 9.1) showed a mass lesion in the left posterior and medial frontal lobe measuring $4.7 \times 3.5 \times 3.5$ cm. The lesion was

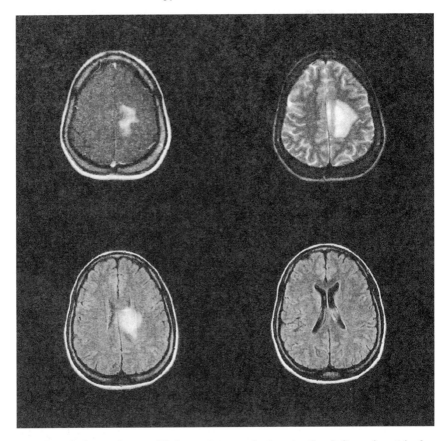

Fig. 9.1. Solitary, large, T2 hyperintense lesion in the left periventricular white matter. Note inhomogeneous pattern of T2 lesion (right upper image).

hypo-intense on T1-weighted images prior to gadolinium administration, hyperintense on T2-weighted sequences, and there was prominent central enhancement on T1-weighted images following gadolinium administration (Fig. 9.2). There was slight effacement and some depression of the left lateral ventricle adjacent to the lesion.

A stereotactic brain biopsy of the left frontal lobe lesion was done on the 13th hospital day.

*   *   *

Discussion

Biopsies from the left frontal lobe consisted of segments of both gray and white matter tissue. Gray matter tissue appeared histologically unremarkable. The white matter showed focal areas of demyelination evident with

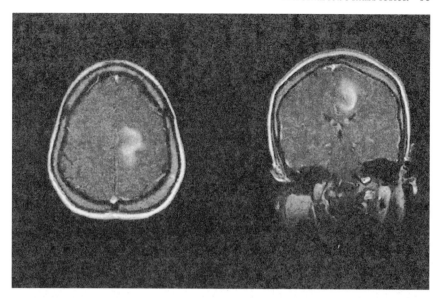

Fig. 9.2. Diffuse enhancement of lesion shown in Fig. 9.1 following administration of gadolinium.

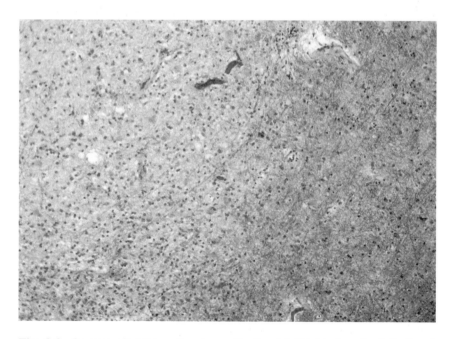

Fig. 9.3. An area of white matter demyelination highlighted on the left. (Luxol fast blue myelin stain, original magnification 200×)

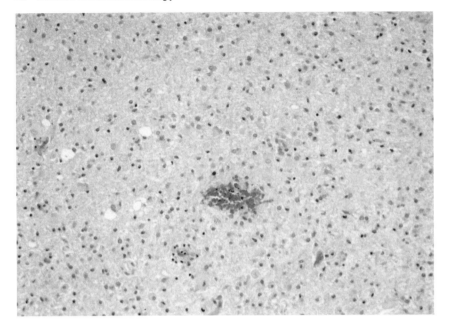

Fig. 9.4. Hypercellular white matter, consisting primarily of macrophages, reactive astrocytes and rare perivascular lymphocytes. (Hematoxylin and eosin, original magnification 200×.)

luxol fast blue stain (Fig. 9.3). These areas were marked histologically by a macrophage infiltrate, reactive astrocytosis, and perivascular chronic inflammation consisting primarily of lymphocytes and macrophages (Fig. 9.4). The majority of the lymphocytes were T cells, because they stained positively for CD3. A smaller population of B lymphocytes (CD20 positive cells) were intermixed with T cells. The area of demyelination was sharply demarcated from adjacent, uninvolved parenchyma. There were no Alzheimer type I astrocytes or viral inclusions. There were no malignant astrocytic cells, and there was no mitotic activity, vascular proliferation, or necrosis to suggest neoplasm. The findings were consistent with inflammatory demyelination.

She was treated with high doses of methylprednisolone followed by oral prednisone in a tapering dose schedule. She gradually improved with intensive rehabilitation, and was fully independent when seen in early November 1999. Repeat MRI showed considerable reduction in the size of the left parietal lesion but the lesion continued to show some enhancement with gadolinium. Also, some surrounding edema persisted. She is being followed.

The differential diagnosis at first included tumor, granulomatous disease, infection, or inflammatory demyelination. There were no granulomas or viral inclusions in the brain biopsy to suggest an infectious etiology. Radiographically, the possibility of a tumor was raised, but histologic features of neoplasm were not present. In particular, there was no evidence of a glioma or atypical features of the lymphoid infiltrate to suggest lymphoma. The constellation of light microscopic findings – white matter macrophages, perivascular chronic inflammation, and reactive astrocytosis – is characteristic of inflammatory demyelination. Similar radiographic and histologic findings have been described by Kepes under the rubric of 'large focal tumor-like demyelinating lesion of the brain.'[1]

The clinical course, MRI findings, CSF findings, and histologic features are most consistent with a monophasic cerebral demyelinating syndrome. Cranial MRI findings in typical MS appear as areas of high signal on T2-weighted images in the cerebral white matter. Characteristically, lesions are seen within the body of the corpus callosum, and extend from the corpus callosum like fingers reaching into the adjacent cerebral white matter. Solitary or confluent nodular lesions occur near or contiguous with the lateral ventricles, and more peripherally in the cerebral white matter. Lesions are also seen in subcortical white matter, in the brainstem and cerebellum, and in the cervical and thoracic spinal cord. The fluid atte-nuated inversion recovery (FLAIR) technique suppresses signal from CSF spaces, increasing the visibility of T2 hyperintense lesions. This provides better visualization of cortical and juxta-cortical lesions; and periventricu-lar lesions are more easily differentiated from ventricular structures. Following administration of gadolinium, T1-weighted images reveal bright, enhancing lesions that represent acute inflammatory lesions. These lesions arise in previously normal white matter, or within areas of T2 lesions, persist for 4–8 weeks, and then subside. Enhancing lesions come and go with variable frequency, but occur much more often than clinical relapses. This patient clearly did not have the typical MRI lesions seen in MS patients.

Kepes[1] described 31 patients with 'large focal tumor-like demyelinating lesion of the brain.' Twenty-four of the 31 patients had solitary lesions, one of which (case 12) had a location, appearance, and clinical features similar to the current case. The initial impression was that of solitary brain tumor in all cases. In each patient, a biopsy showed inflammatory demye-lination, as in this patient. Three of the 31 patients developed additional lesions consistent with MS during follow-up, but it was unclear how consistently the patients were followed. Kepes suggested that the tumor-like demyelinating lesions might share features with both multiple sclerosis and acute disseminated encephalomyelitis.

The relationship between tumor-like demyelinating lesions and MS is uncertain. Weinshenker and Lucchinetti[2] reviewed the differential diagnosis of 'acute leukoencephalopathies,' which included acute transverse myelitis, acute disseminated encephalomyelitis (ADEM), acute progressive MS (Marburg disease), neuromyelitis optica (Devic disease), recurrent myelitis, and focal cerebral demyelination (which Kepes termed 'tumor-like demyelinating lesion'). Weinshenker and Lucchinetti suggested that these conditions may be variations of autoimmune inflammatory demyelinating diseases, because they have all have been reported to respond to steroid therapy, and because initially monophasic disorders such as ADEM or transverse myelitis may subsequently relapse and remit in a pattern typical of MS. Even though the clinical and pathologic features of these conditions overlap, it is still unclear whether they are etiologically distinct entities, or phenotypic variations of one disease.

Diagnosis

Inflammatory demyelination.

References

1. Kepes JJ. Large focal tumor-like demyelinating lesions of the brain: intermediate entity between multiple sclerosis and acute disseminated encephalomyelitis? A study of 31 patients [see comments]. *Ann Neurol* 1993; **33:** 18–27.
2. Weinshenker B, Lucchinetti C. Acute leukoencephalopathies: differential diagnosis and investigation. *Neurologist* 2000; **4:** 148–166.

Spontaneous low pressure headache

Clinical history and examination

A 30-year-old woman developed the sudden onset of a severe orthostatic headache while reaching for an object on the ground. A mild headache, which she rated as a 2 on a 10-point intensity scale, persisted when she was recumbent, and she developed a 9/10 headache and posterior neck pain upon standing. When she maintained an upright position, she developed nausea and vomiting. Severe neck pain and headache were precipitated by cough or straining. In addition, the patient experienced intrascapular pain, radicular pain that radiated to the left arm, and an occasional sensation of distorted hearing.

The patient had no prior headache history. She did not have chest pain, shortness of breath, sore throat, diarrhea, fever, rash, or arthralgias. She presented to the neurologist after being symptomatic for 1 month. She appeared ill and uncomfortable. General and neurologic examinations were otherwise normal. She did not have a stiff neck.

Investigations were undertaken.

Magnetic resonance imaging (MRI) of the brain revealed descent of the cerebellar tonsils 4 mm below the foramen magnum. Diffuse pachymeningeal hyperintensity was found after gadolinium. Lumbar puncture revealed an opening pressure of 20 mm of cerebrospinal fluid (CSF), a pleocytosis of 40 WBC, and a slightly elevated CSF protein of 85 mg/dl with a normal glucose. The patient was treated conservatively with bedrest, hydration, several boluses of intravenous caffeine, and oral theophylline, but there was no improvement. After 1 week a radioisotope cisternogram demonstrated rapid clearance of the radioisotope but no leak was found. Computed tomography (CT) myelogram demonstrated extravasation of contrast from a nerve sleeve diverticuleum at left C7.

*   *   *

Discussion

The patient was diagnosed with low pressure headache due to a torn nerve root sleeve. Spontaneous CSF leaks are rare. The true incidence and prevalence of this disorder are not known. The Mayo Clinic series of 39 patients with spontaneous low CSF pressure headache had an equal representation of men and women.[1] It was first described by Schaltenbrand,[2] a German neurologist, who termed it 'aliquorrhea.' In the USA, spontaneous low CSF pressure with clinical features resembling a post-lumbar headache was first described by Henry Woltman.[3] Because headache is common and the neurologic examination is normal, this syndrome is underrecognized. Lay et al.[1] believe that most cases of spontaneous low CSF pressure headache are caused by CSF leaks.

Headache is the most common clinical symptom of intracranial hypotension. It is accentuated when the patient assumes the erect position and relieved when he or she assumes the recumbent position (orthostatic headache). In a large series of 239 patients with post-lumbar headache, which is felt to have a headache pattern identical to spontaneous low pressure headache, the time to headache onset on standing varied from immediate to 265 minutes (median 20 seconds). The time to maximal headache ranged from 30 seconds to 60 minutes (median 30 seconds) and the time to headache relief, on lying down, varied from 0 to 15 minutes (median 20 seconds). The severity of the headache was negatively correlated with the time the headache started or reached its maximum but did not correlate with the time to resolution on lying down.[4] The headache of spontaneous low CSF pressure is usually bilateral and generalized, frontal, or occipital. It is typically exacerbated by head movement, coughing, straining, sneezing, or jugular vein compression. Pain may be associated with one or more of the following: nausea, emesis, pain or tight feeling of the neck, intrascapular pain, dizziness, diplopia (usually a horizontal diplopia related to unilateral or bilateral sixth nerve palsy), photophobia, distorted hearing, blurred vision, superior binasal visual field defects, radicular upper limb symptoms, and (rarely) facial numbness or weakness.[5] A slow or vagus pulse has been described.[6] Mokri[5] has broadened the clinical spectrum by describing patients with a constant lingering headache that only worsened slightly when the patient assumed the upright position. Some people with low CSF pressure do not develop headache[7] (Table 10.1). A distinction must be made between a patient with an orthostatic headache that is relieved by recumbency and a patient with a headache that is aggravated by movement or by assuming the upright posture.

Intracranial hypotension can be divided into two categories: (1) spontaneous intracranial hypotension with no evidence of CSF leak or systemic illness, and (2) symptomatic intracranial hypotension, which may be associated with a CSF leak.[6] A low CSF pressure headache is classified as one that 'occurs or worsens less than 15 minutes after assuming the

Table 10.1. Features of low CSF pressure headache.

Pain
  – aggravated by upright position
  – relieved with recumbency
  – aggravated by head shaking and jugular compression
Associated symptoms
  – anorexia
  – blurry vision
  – diplopia
  – dizziness
  – generalized malaise
  – interscapular pain
  – nausea
  – photophobia
  – tinnitus
  – vomiting
Physical examination
  – within normal limits
  – rare neck stiffness, slow pulse rate ('vagus pulse')
  – rare sixth nerve palsy

upright position and disappears or improves less than 30 minutes after resuming the recumbent position.'[8]

The most common cause of intracranial hypotension is lumbar puncture, whether done diagnostically (e.g. for myelography) or for anesthesia. Head or back trauma, craniotomy, and spinal surgery can produce CSF hypotension as a result of a dural tear or a traumatic avulsion of a nerve root that results in a CSF leak.[9–11] Low-pressure syndromes also occur as a result of CSF rhinorrhea, whether spontaneous, post-traumatic, or caused by a pituitary tumor. Cerebrospinal fluid hypotension can be caused by a systemic medical illness, including severe dehydration, hyperpnea, meningoencephalitis, a severe systemic infection, or uremia, or by infusion of hypertonic solution. Other causes of positional headache, such as a colloid cyst of the third ventricle, need to be ruled out[12] (Table 10.2).

When intracranial hypotension is present, intracranial CSF pressure falls more when the upright posture is assumed. This produces increased traction on the supporting structures of the brain, and traction on these pain-sensitive structures (blood vessels and dural sinuses) may cause headache in the upright position. Secondary compensatory venous dilation may contribute to the headache as well.[13,14] No direct correlation exists between the level of pressure on a subsequent lumbar puncture and the presence of low-pressure (as well as high-pressure) headache, but a correlation exists between CSF volume loss and headache.[15,16] Using

Table 10.2. Causes of low-pressure headache syndrome.

Spontaneous intracranial hypotension
Symptomatic
  Lumbar puncture: diagnostic, myelographic, and spinal anesthesia
  Traumatic: head or back trauma
    – with CSF leak: dural tear, traumatic nerve root avulsion
    – without CSF leak
  Postoperative: craniotomy, spinal surgery, post pneumonectomy
    (thoracoarachnoid fistula)
    – with CSF leak
    – without CSF leak
  Malfunctioning CSF shunt
  Spontaneous CSF leak: CSF rhinorrhea, occult pituitary tumor, dural tear
  Systemic illnesses: dehydration, diabetic coma, hyperpnea,
    meningoencephalitis, uremia, severe systemic infection

MRI, Iqbal et al.[17] demonstrated that CSF usually leaks into the paraspinous area after a lumbar puncture, but the severity of the post-lumbar puncture headache does not correlate with the volume of the escaped fluid. Jugular compression increases the severity of headache despite increasing intracranial pressure, suggesting that the headache is not caused solely by intracranial hypotension.[15]

Grant and associates found no change in the position of the intracranial structures in patients with intracranial hypotension.[16] Other workers, however, have found downward displacement of the brain with incisural or cerebellar tonsillar herniation, which could be mistaken for a Chiari malformation.[18–20] In the Mayo Clinic series, 62% of the 26 patients had evidence of descent of the brain. This included Chiari I malformation (cerebellar descent), reduction in size or effacement of the prepontine cistern, inferior displacement of the optic chiasm, effacement or obliteration of the perichiasmatic cisterns, and descent of the iter.[1] The downward displacement might have been worse if an upright scan had been performed. These MRI abnormalities often resolve with headache improvement or treatment.[18,21] Thus, headache may result from either painful venous dilation or displacement of and traction on pain-sensitive intracranial structures.

Occult CSF leakage is probably the major cause of spontaneous intracranial hypotension.[22–24] A history of minor trauma is often elicited.[25] In 39 Mayo Clinic cases, 52% had a history of minor trauma or an inciting event. These included falling onto the buttocks,[26,27] a sudden twist or stretch,[22,28,29] sexual intercourse or orgasm,[29] a sudden sneeze or paroxysmal coughing,[30] vigorous exercise,[31] or strenuous effort during racket sports.[32] Traumatic rupture of spinal epidural cysts (formed during development), perineural cysts, or a nerve sheath tear[19,22,23,25,26,32,33] could

Table 10.3. Paraclinical findings in persistent headache.

1. Reduced CSF opening pressure from 0 to 65 mm CSF in the lateral decubitus position
2. CSF pleocytosis and increased protein concentrations
3. Diffuse pachymeningeal enhancement
4. Subdural collections
5. Slit ventricles with tight basilar cisterns
6. Imaging evidence of descent of the brain
   Secondary Chiari I malformation
   Flattening of basis pontis
   Bowing of the optic chiasm over the pituitary glands
7. Pituitary engorgemant

produce a cryptic CSF leak. Cerebrospinal fluid can also leak into the petrous or ethmoidal regions or through the cribriform plate. The patient may swallow the fluid and be unaware of the leak.

Paraclinical findings in low pressure headache are catalogued in Table 10.3. The opening pressure may be zero or even negative. It is usually less than 70 mmH$_2$O; however, patients with the clinical and radiologic findings of low pressure headache but normal CSF pressure have been described.[34] CSF pleocytosis and increased protein are thought to be due to diapedesis of cells and leakage of protein from related meningeal veins.

MRI with gadolinium is more useful than CT in evaluating patients with low-pressure headache. Diffuse pachymeningeal enhancement (Fig. 10.1a,b) is common on gadolinium-enhanced MRI.[1] Before diffuse meningeal enhancement was a recognized feature of low-pressure headache, patients often had extensive testing to rule out other causes of diffuse meningeal enhancement such as carcinomatosis, meningitis, and sarcoidosis.[35] The presence of diffuse meningeal enhancement in the clinical setting of an orthostatic headache is strongly suggestive of low pressure headache. Diffuse pachymeningeal enhancement involves both the supratentorial and infratentorial compartments, surrounding the brain without abnormal enhancement in the sulci or around the brainstem.[19,35,36] Diffuse pachymeningeal enhancement has shown inflammatory changes in some, but not in other, pathologic studies.[23,37] It improves or resolves with headache resolution. Descent of the brain may accompany low pressure headache. Findings include cerebellar tonsilar herniation (Fig. 10.2), descent of the brainstem, descent of the basis pontis, and partial bowing of the optic chiasm.[19,36–38] These findings may resolve with headache resolution.

Subdural hematomas or hygromas have been observed to result from low intracranial pressure.[2] The subdural hematomas are presumably caused by rupture of bridging veins as the brain sags.[2] MRI of the spine may be useful to identify CSF leaks.

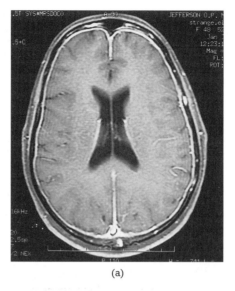

(a)

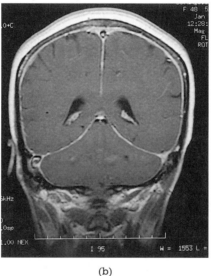

(b)

Fig. 10.1. Diffuse pachymeningeal hyperintensity after gadolinium-enhanced MRI (two views in the same patient).

Radioisotope cisternography is useful for identifying CSF leaks.[39] Cotton pledgets are placed in the nasopharynx and marked according to their position. A radioisotope tracer is placed in the lumbar CSF space or via a cervicocisternal tap. Serial images are obtained at 2, 6, 24, and sometimes 48 hours. The pledgets are then taken out and checked for tracer. Findings may include CSF hyperabsorption or leak with early clearance and premature appearance of tracer in the bladder and

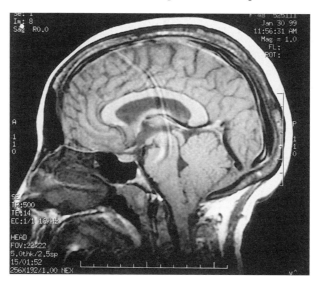

Fig. 10.2. Magnetic resonance imaging scan demonstrating descent of the cerebellar tonsils through the foramen magnum.

kidneys. A leak in the spine may also be demonstrated. Radioactivity of the pledgets identifies a CSF leak through the cribriform plate and partially localizes the leak based upon which pledget has the maximum radioactivity.

In order to identify the source of a CSF leak, a CT myelogram may be necessary. It may show arachnoid diverticula of spinal roots with or without CSF loss. A 'dump study' involves tipping a patient during a myelogram to allow dye to enter the cranial CSF spaces. A CT may identify leakage through the cribriform plate or other skull defect.

Treatment

Treatment of low CSF pressure headache begins with noninvasive, non-pharmacologic therapeutic modalities (Table 10.4) that include bed-rest, hydration, and an abdominal binder. This treatment is not cost-effective if it is prolonged, however. If there is no improvement, intravenous or oral pharmacologic therapy beginning with caffeine may produce significant relief. Methylxanthines (caffeine, theophylline) decrease cerebral blood flow and increase cerebral vascular resistance. They also increase CSF production by stimulating the sodium–potassium pumps.[40]

Intravenous and oral caffeine has been used to treat post-lumbar puncture headaches for 50 years. In a controlled double-blind prospective study, Sechzer and Abel[41] showed that 500 mg of caffeine sodium benzoate given intravenously was dramatically effective in 75% of patients with low CSF pressure who had undergone a previous lumbar puncture. A second

Table 10.4. Treatment of low-CSF headache.

Nonpharmacologic
  Bed-rest
  Abdominal binder
Intravenous and oral pharmacologic
  Caffeine, theophylline
  Corticosteroids, ACTH
Epidural interventions
  Blood patch
  Sodium chloride
  Dextran patch
  Morphine sulphate

---

dose, given after two hours, raised the success rate to 85%. Jarvis et al.,[42] in an open study, used 2 liters of intravenous Ringer's lactate solution: the first, given over 1 hour, contained 500 mg of caffeine sodium benzoate.[41] The second was given over 2 hours. Both could be repeated after 4 hours. The total response rate in 18 patients was 75%.[42]

A placebo-controlled, double-blind study of 300 mg of oral caffeine (120% of the dose of caffeine in caffeine sodium benzoate (250 mg caffeine, 250 mg sodium benzoate)) was performed in 40 postpartum patients. Beneficial effects were obtained rapidly, with relief occurring within 4 hours in 70% of patients, and without symptom recurrence.[43]

Theophylline, available in oral and parenteral forms, has also been used for low-pressure headache. In a placebo-controlled, double-blind pilot study, Feuerstein and Zeides treated 11 patients with post-lumbar puncture headache with either oral theophylline (281.7 mg) or placebo three times a day.[44] Theophylline treatment allowed patients to sit up for a 30-minute period sooner than without the treatment. Kasner et al.[21] found it to be effective in a patient whose spontaneous intracranial hypotension did not respond to a blood patch.

A brief trial of steroids in combination with bed-rest, an abdominal binder, or caffeine can be beneficial. If no relief is obtained within 24 hours, a quick steroid taper is recommended because of potential side-effects. ACTH 1.5 units/kg in 1–2 liters of lactated Ringers solution with a possible repeat dose in 24 hours has been reported to be effective.[40]

Epidural administration of agents is indicated if the patient continues to be symptomatic after a noninvasive medical approach. This was originally thought to work by providing a plug or seal to the dural tear. The epidural blood patch (originally described by Gormley[45] is the most successful reported treatment (96.8% success rate) and the most frequently used procedure for low CSF pressure headache.[45–48] It is performed by infusing 10–20 ml of autologous blood into the epidural space under sterile conditions. A prospective study conducted to evaluate the efficacy of different volumes of blood found no difference between 10 ml and 10–15 ml of blood (determined by patient height). The blood patch was initially successful in 91% of patients 2 hours after the procedure. In the long term, 87% of patients were satisfied, but only 61% had both immediate and permanent relief. The volume that was injected made no difference.[49] Many investigators have performed blood patches for spontaneous intracranial hypotension and have described similar results.

The presumed mechanism of action of the blood patch is an immediate gelatinous tamponade of a dural leak followed by fibrin deposition and fibroblastic activity. The blood patch can tolerate a pressure as high as 40 mm of mercury soon after coagulation.[49] Collagen deposition and scar formation are complete within 3 weeks. This mechanism has recently been challenged, however, by several investigators who have noted recurrence of orthostatic headache 4–6 months after a successful blood patch.[50] They propose that compression of the dural sac with an increment in CSF pressure may serve as a signal that deactivates the low CSF pressure headache, possibly by antagonizing adenosine receptors.[50] However, Usubiaga and associates monitored epidural and subarachnoid pressure changes in 24 patients.[51] Injection of 10–20 ml of saline into the epidural space produced a transient (3–10 minutes) rise in pressure in both spaces. The authors of the paper believe that the brief increase in pressure could not account for the prolonged headache relief and the saline injection promoted the development of a fibrin clot.

The extradural blood patch, when examined by MRI at 30 minutes and 3 hours, has a mass effect that compresses the dural sac and displaces the conus medullaris and cauda equina. The main bulk of the clot occupied four or five vertebral levels, with a thinner spread cephalad and caudad. Some blood initially entered the CSF, changing the MRI signal, but this had concentrated to a focal dural clot by 3 hours. After 7 hours the mass effect had disappeared.[52] If the headache of intracranial hypotension recurs, a repeat blood patch can be performed.

A retrospective study of 196 patients treated with the epidural blood patch revealed no major complications; 37% had pain at the site of injection, 12% had leg pain, 10% had sensory disturbances in the lower extremities, 8% had gait disturbance, and 8% had leg weakness. These symptoms were mild and transient.[53]

Alternative epidural treatments are available for those patients who fail the blood patch, have suspected sepsis, are HIV positive, or refuse to use blood products. Epidural 0.9% sodium chloride solution has been used in boluses of 30–50 ml since first described by Rice and Dobbs.[54] Baysinger et al.[55] used a bolus of 30–50 ml of epidural sodium chloride 0.9% followed by continuous infusion at a rate of 25–30 ml/h for 24 hours to successfully treat two patients who failed at least three epidural blood patches. Others have used intermittent boluses of 10–30 ml, which could be repeated every 3–4 hours.[51] Continuous intrathecal saline infusion requires an epidural catheter placed at the L-2/3 level. Saline infusion at a rate of

20–30 ml/h can be initiated by a bolus of saline and can be continued up to 72 hours.[47,56]

Epidural dextran, which is slowly absorbed from the epidural space, has been used to treat post-lumbar puncture headache. Barrios-Alarcon et al.[57] used 20–30 mg of epidural dextran 40 (1–1.5 ml for every 10 cm of height). There was no recurrence in 64% of the patients on long-term follow-up. Other authors support the use of epidural dextran but state that its safety and efficacy need to be compared to the epidural blood patch.[40] Eldor et al.[58] suggest the use of epidural morphine, based on anecdotal experience. It could be the morphine itself or the volume of fluid in which it is contained that contributes to pain relief. Epidural morphine is not a routine treatment for post-lumbar puncture headache at this time.

Diagnosis

Low pressure headache.

References

1. Lay CL, Campbell JK, Mokri B. Low cerebrospinal fluid pressure headache. In: Goadsby PJ, Silberstein SD, eds. *Headache*. Boston: Butterworth-Heinemann, 1997: 355–368.
2. Schaltenbrand G. Neure Anschauen zor Pathophysiologie der Liquorzirkulation. *Zentralb Nforchir* 1938; **3**: 290–300.
3. Woltman HW. Headache: a consideration of some of the more common types. *Med Clin N Am*, 1940; **24**: 1159–1170.
4. Vilming ST, Kloster R. Postlumbar puncture headache: clinical features and suggestions for diagnostic criteria. *Cephalalgia* 1997; **17**: 778–784.
5. Mokri B 1999 Spontaneous CSF leaks: from intracranial hypotension to CSF hypovolemia – evolution of a concept. *Mayo Clin Proc* 1999; **74**: 1113–23.
6. Marcelis J, Silberstein SD. Spontaneous low cerebrospinal fluid pressure headache. *Headache* 1990; **30**: 192–6.
7. Marshall J. Lumbar-puncture headache. *J Neurol Neurosurg Psychiatry* 1950; **13**: 71.
8. Headache Classification Committee of the International Headache Society. Classification and diagnostic criteria for headache disorders, cranial neuralgia, and facial pain. *Cephalalgia* 1988; **8**: 1–96.
9. Kieffer SA, Wolff JM, Prentice WB et al. Scinticisternography in individuals without known neurological disease. *Am J Roentgenology* 1971; **112**: 236.
10. Front D, Penning L. Subcutaneous extravasation of CSF demonstration by scinticisternography. *Nuclear Med* 1973; **15**: 200–201.
11. Sharrock NE. Postural headache following thoracic somatic paravertebral nerve block. *Anesthesiology* 1980; **52**: 360–362.
12. Young WB, Silberstein SD. Paroxysmal headache caused by colloid cyst of the third ventricle: case report and review of the literature. *Headache* 1997; **37**: 15–20.
13. Dalessio DJ. *Wolff's Headache and other Head Pain*. Oxford: Oxford University Press, 1972.
14. Cass W, Edelist G. Post spinal headache. *JAMA* 1974; **227**: 786–787.

15. Raskin NH. Lumbar puncture headache: a review. *Headache* 1990; **30:** 197–200.
16. Grant R, Condon B, Hart I et al. Changes in intracranial CSF volume after lumbar puncture and their relationship to post-LP headache. *J Neurol Neurosurg Psychiatry*, 1991; **54:** 440–442.
17. Iqbal J, Davis LE, Orrison WW. An MRI study of lumbar puncture headaches. *Headache* 1995; **35:** 420–422.
18. Pannullo S, Reich J, Posner J. Meningeal enhancement associated with low intracranial pressure. *Neurology* 1992; **42:** 430.
19. Fishman RA, Dillon WP. Dural enhancement and cerebral displacement secondary to intracranial hypotension. *Neurology* 1993; **43:** 609–611.
20. Good DC, Ghobrial M. Pathologic changes associated with intracranial hypotension and meningeal enhancement on MRI. *Neurology*, 1993; **43:** 2698–2700.
21. Kasner SE, Rosenfield J, Farber RE. Spontaneous intracranial hypotension: headache with a reversible Arnold–Chiari malformation. *Headache*, 1995; **35:** 557–559.
22. Lasater GM. Primary intracranial hypotension. *Headache*, 1970; **10:** 63–66.
23. Rando TA, Fishman RA. Spontaneous intracranial hypotension: report of two cases and review of the literature. *Neurology* 1992; **42:** 481–487.
24. Schievink WI, Meyer FB, Atkinson JL et al. Spontaneous spinal cerebrospinal fluid leaks and intracranial hypotension. *J Neurosurg* 1996; **84:** 598–605.
25. Lake AP, Minckler J, Scanlan RL. Spinal epidural cyst: theories of pathogenesis. *J Neurosurg* 1974; **40:** 774–778.
26. Nosik WA. Intracranial hypotension secondary to lumbar nerve sleeve tear. *JAMA* 1955; **157:** 1110–1111.
27. Bell WE, Joynt RJ, Sahs AL. Low spinal fluid pressure syndromes. *Neurology* 1958; **8:** 157–163.
28. Horton JC, Fishman RA. Neurovisual findings in the syndrome of spontaneous intracranial hypotension from aural cerebrospinal fluid leak. *Ophthalmology* 1994 **101:** 244–251.
29. Paulson GW, Klawans HL. Benign orgasmic cephalalgia. *Headache* 1974; **13:** 181–187.
30. Baker CC. Headache due to spontaneous low spinal fluid pressure. *Minn Med* 1983; **66:** 325–328.
31. Capobianco DJ, Kuczler FJ. Case report: primary intracranial hypotension. *Nilit Med* 1990; **155:** 64–66.
32. Garcia-Albea E, Cabrera F, Tejeiro J et al. Delayed postexertional headache, intracranial hypotension and racket sports (letter). *J Neurol Neurosurg Psychiatry*, 1992; **55:** 975.
33. Ferraraccio BE. Positional headache due to spontaneous intracranial hypotension (letter). *South Med J* 1992; **85:** 47.
34. Mokri B, Hunter SF, Atkinson JL et al. Orthostatic headaches caused by CSF leak but with normal CSF pressures. *Neurology* 1998; **51:** 786–790.
35. Hochman MS, Naidich TP, Kobetz SA et al. Spontaneous intracranial hypotension with pachymeningeal enhancement on MRI. *Neurology* 1992; **42:** 1628–1630.
36. Sable SG, Ramadan NM. Meningeal enhancement and low CSF pressure headache. An MRI study. *Cephalalgia* 1991; **11:** 275–276.
37. Mokri B, Parisi JE, Scheithauer BW et al. Meningeal biopsy in intracranial hypotension: meningeal enhancement on MRI. *Neurology* 1995; **45:** 1801–1807.

38. Murros K, Fogelholm R. Spontaneous intracranial hypotension with slit ventricles. *J Neurol Neurosurg Psychiatry* 1983; **46:** 1149–1151.
39. Molins A, Alvarez J, Somalla J et al. Cisternographic pattern of spontaneous liquoral hypotension. *Cephalalgia* 1990; **10:** 59–65.
40. Choi A, Laurito CE, Cunningham FE. Pharmacologic management of postdural puncture headache. *Ann Pharmacother* 1996; **30:** 831–839.
41. Sechzer PH, Abel L. Post-spinal anesthesia headache treated with caffeine. *Curr Therapeutic Res* 1978; **24;** 307–312.
42. Jarvis AP, Greenawalt JW, Fagraeus L. *Anesth Analg* 1986; **65:** 313–321.
43. Camann WR, Murray RS, Mushlin PS et al. Effects of oral caffeine on postdural puncture headache. *Anesth Analg* 1990; **70:** 181–184.
44. Feuerstein TJ, Zeides A. Theophylline relieves headache following lumbar puncture: placebo-controlled, double-blind pilot study. *Klinische Wochenschrift* 1986; **64:** 216–218.
45. Gormley JB. Treatment of post-spinal headache. *Anesthesiology* 1960; **21:** 565–566.
46. Ostheimer GW, Palahniuk RJ, Shnider SM. Epidural blood patch for post-lumbar-puncture headache. *Anesthesiology* 1974; **41:** 307–308.
47. Bart AJ, Wheeler AS. Comparison of epidural saline infusion and epidural blood placement in the treatment of post lumbar puncture headache. *Anesthesiology* 1978; **48:** 221–223.
48. Millette PC, Paqacz A, Charest C. Epidural blood patch for the treatment of chronic headache after myelography. *Journal de l'Association Canadienne des Radiologistes* 1982; **33:** 236–238.
49. Taivainen T, Pitkanen M, Tuominen M et al. Efficacy of epidural blood patch for postdural puncture headache. *Acta Anaesthesiol Scand* 1993; **37:** 702–705.
50. Raskin NH. Headache. New York: Churchill-Livingstone, 1988.
51. Usubiaga JE, Usubiaga LE, Brea LM et al. Epidural and subarachnoid space pressures and relation to postspinal anesthesia headache. *Anesth Analg* 1967; **46:** 293–296.
52. Beards SC, Jackson A, Griffiths AG et al. Magnetic resonance imaging of extradural blood patches: appearances from 30 min to 18 h. *Anesthesiology* 1993; **71:** 182–188.
53. Tarkkila PJ, Miralles JA, Palomaki EA. The subjective complications and efficiency of the epidural blood patch in the treatment of postdural puncture headache. *Reg Anaesth* 1989; **14:** 247–250.
54. Rice CG, Dobbs CH. The use of peridural and subarachnoid injections of saline solutions in the treatment of severe postspinal headache. *Anesthesiology* 1950; **11:** 17–23.
55. Baysinger CL, Menk EJ, Harte E et al. The successful treatment of dural puncture headache after failed epidural blood patch. *Anesth Analg* 1986; **65:** 1242–1244.
56. Peterson RC, Freeman DP, Knox CA, Gibson BE. Successful treatment of spontaneous low cerebrospinal fluid pressure headache. *Ann Neurol* 1987; **22:** 148 (Abstract).
57. Barrios-Alarcon J, Aldrete JA, Paragas-Tapia D. Relief of post-lumbar puncture headache with epidural dextran 40: a preliminary report. *Reg Anesth* 1989; **14:** 78–80.
58. Eldor J, Burstein M, Guedj P. Spinal morphine injections for treatment of postspinal headache. *J Anesthesiol* 1992; **6:** 507–509.

A 23-year-old man with arm and vocal tremor

Clinical history and examination

A 23-year-old man presented with a 7-year history of arm and vocal tremor. A proficient French horn player, he first noted a deterioration in his playing at the age of 16. He developed a tremor when attempting to sustain long tones and had difficulty maintaining airflow into the mouthpiece of the instrument. Mild tremor of the left hand interfered with his ability to depress the stops on the horn. Although he enrolled in a major conservatory at the age of 18, he was unable to maintain an acceptable standard of playing and was forced to leave school. His symptoms were attributed to the stress of performance.

By age 21, his left-hand tremor became more noticeable, and it began to interfere with other fine motor activities. Present only with action and posture, it never occurred at rest. A similar but less intense tremor soon affected the left and then the right leg. His gait changed as well with mild unsteadiness, and he experienced a slight tremor of his head when walking. Treatment with primidone and propranolol did not improve his symptoms. Consumption of alcohol and treatment with clonazepam 0.5 mg b.i.d. did symptomatically improve his arm tremor but did not eliminate it.

Review of the patient's family history revealed no history of parental consanguinity. His mother was of Sicilian and Ukrainian extraction, and his father came from French and Ukrainian heritage. No other first-degree relative had neurologic complaints except for his brother. At the age of 13, he developed a very mild tremor of his hands, which slightly interfered with writing and drinking. His deficits were so mild, however, that he was able to pursue a degree in architecture. There was no history of arm tremor at rest, no change in his speech and no voice tremor. His medical history was notable for several episodes of hematuria occurring during contact sports, a history of kidney stones, and a slightly enlarged spleen.

Neurologic examination of our patient was notable for dysarthric, scanning and slightly slow speech accompanied by a vocal tremor of approximately 3 Hz. Aside from mild depression, his mental status was normal. There was no facial masking or risorius grin. Motor examination revealed mild hypotonia without cogwheeling or bradykinesia. A 3 Hz proximal wingbeating tremor was present on posture and action, affecting the left side more than the right, more severe in the arms than the legs. Rapid alternating movements were mildly uncoordinated, with dysdiadochokinesis and dysmetria. His gait was normal in stance and stride, with very mild head titubation triggered by walking. Sensory modalities and reflexes were normal. There was no parkinsonism or extremity dystonia.

Routine laboratory studies revealed a platelet count of 100 k (normal 165–415). Total bilirubin (2.7 mg/dl, normal 0.30–1.30) and direct bilirubin (0.8 mg/dl, normal 0.04–0.38) were mildly elevated. The remainder of the routine chemistry and hematology studies were normal. An abdominal ultrasound revealed mild hepatomegaly and marked splenomegaly.

*   *   *

Discussion

This 23-year-old man presented with a 7-year history of tremor affecting the voice, arms and legs. Tremor, best defined as an 'involuntary, appropriately rhythmic and roughly sinusoidal movement,'[1] is the most common movement disorder. It is usually easily distinguished from other movement disorders, although irregular jerky tremors may mimic myoclonus. The most common cause of tremor in the adult population is essential tremor.[2] Often inherited in an autosomal dominant pattern, patients with essential tremor have tremor without other neurologic signs. Essential tremor most commonly affects the hands, and also frequently affects the head and voice. Involvement of the legs is exceedingly rare. More common in older patients, essential tremor may affect people of all ages. Typically 6 Hz in frequency, it is primarily a kinetic tremor affecting the wrist and fingers. Spread of tremor to rest is not uncommon, particularly in more severe cases or when tremor has been present for a long time. Although usually slowly progressive, patients may become completely disabled from tremor. Treatment with propranolol and/or primidone often produces moderate symptomatic improvement, although side-effects often limit the use of these agents.[2]

It is usually not difficult to differentiate essential tremor from other disorders that cause kinetic tremor. Physiologic tremor, an 8–12 Hz tremor present during maintenance of limb posture, is seen in normal individuals and is typically enhanced by sleep deprivation, stress and excess caffeine intake.[1] Its fine amplitude and episodic appearance usually help distinguish it from pathologic tremor states. A wide variety of drugs and toxins can also cause tremor. Among these agents, lithium and valproic acid are the two most common offenders, producing a clinical profile that can be indistinguishable from essential tremor.

Cerebellar tremor is another important cause of kinetic tremor. Typically slower in frequency (3–5 Hz), cerebellar tremor may affect the extremities and the trunk, often producing a characteristic vertical oscillation of the head called titubation. Usually slower than the frequency of essential tremor, cerebellar tremor is nearly always accompanied by cerebellar signs, i.e. scanning speech, dysarthria, dysmetria, past-pointing, hypotonia, impaired check and wide-based ataxic gait.

The description of this patient's clinical history and exam are most consistent with a disorder of cerebellar outflow. His tremor was a pure action tremor, affecting arms and voice but also involving his legs on exam. Scanning speech and dysarthria are not consistent with a diagnosis of essential tremor. The diagnosis of a cerebellar disorder was secured by the frequency of his tremor (3 Hz), its proximal nature, and the presence of dysdiadochokinesis and dysmetria, features also not seen in essential tremor. Although his brother also had tremor, onset of tremor in the second decade would be uncommon for essential tremor.

A number of neurodegenerative diseases may present in the first two decades of life with a movement disorder. Patients with these disorders, including the gangliosidoses, Gauchers disease, mucopolysaccharidoses, mitochondrial disorders and others, typically present with an abnormal movement disorder accompanied by global cognitive decline. One neurodegenerative disorder however may present with tremor in relative isolation – Wilsons disease.

The diagnosis of Wilsons disease was made in this patient at the bedside by careful examination of his eyes. By illuminating his irises from the side and varying the angle of the light on the eye, it was possible to see Kayser–Fleischer rings in the outer cornea of both eyes, even though his irises were brown. They extended around the full circumference of the iris, thicker superiorly and inferiorly, and were later documented by slit-lamp examination by an experienced neuro-ophthalmologist. The diagnosis of Wilson's disease was confirmed biochemically by a depression in his serum ceruloplasmin to 8 mg/dl (normal 25–63), low serum copper of 48 μmg/dl (normal 70–155), and an elevated 24-hour urine copper excretion of 62 μmg (normal 15–50). Direct sequencing of the patient's DNA encoding the copper-transporting P-type ATPase ATP7B (the Wilsons disease gene)[3] revealed that he was homozygous for a missense mutation at amino acid 1069 (His to Gln).

An MRI of the head was obtained (Fig. 11.1a–c), revealing increased signal involving the ventrolateral thalamus, posterior limbs of the internal capsule, middle and superior cerebellar peduncles, and splenium and genu of the corpus callosum on T2 and proton-dense images. Mild to moderate atrophy of the midbrain and pons was present as well.

He was treated with penicillamine with gradually increasing doses to 250 mg q.i.d. Marked urine copper excretion (876 µmg/24 h, normal 15–50) was achieved within 2 weeks. Although he was subsequently treated with trientene and zinc, his tremor continued unchanged. After our patient was diagnosed, his brother underwent slit-lamp examination revealing prominent Kayser–Fleischer rings. A diagnosis of Wilsons disease was confirmed biochemically, and he was treated with trientene and zinc.

In 1912, Wilson described the cardinal features of the illness that would later bear his name.[4] Wilsons disease is an inherited autosomal recessive disorder of copper metabolism. The responsible gene encodes the ATP7B protein, a protein that binds copper and assists in its excretion.[3] The fundamental defect in Wilsons disease is an inability to adequately excrete copper. Copper accumulates in the liver where it is stored, instead of being excreted into the gut. It eventually spills into the blood and accumulates in other organs, most notably in the kidneys and brain. Patients may present with hepatic insufficiency, neurologic or psychiatric symptoms, in isolation or combination.[5]

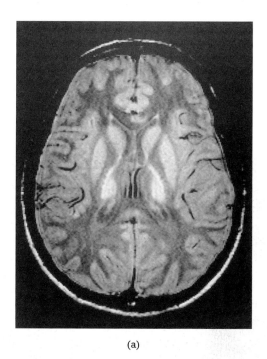

(a)

Fig. 11.1. (a) A proton-dense axial image demonstrates symmetric high signal in the lateral thalamus and posterior limb of the internal capsule in a patient with Wilsons disease. The striatum is spared. (b) A T2 axial image shows high signal in the middle and superior cerebellar peduncles. (c) Sagittal image demonstrates foci of high signal in the splenium and genu of the corpus callosum.

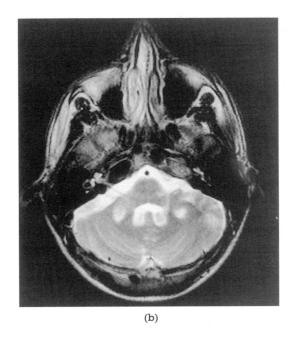

(b)

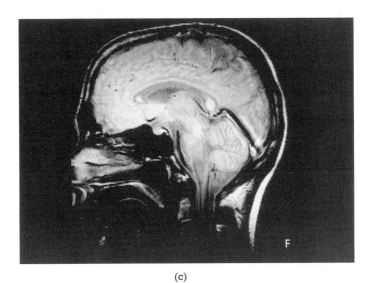

(c)

Fig. 11.1. (*continued*)

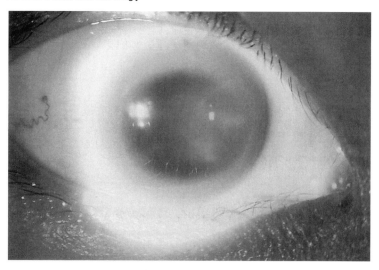

Fig. 11.2. A Kayser–Fleischer ring is present, extending around the full circumference of the cornea.

The diagnosis of Wilsons disease is typically made by documenting the triad of Kayser–Fleischer rings, low serum ceruloplasmin and elevated urinary copper excretion. Serum copper levels are not helpful in the diagnosis. Also, as many as 10% of patients with Wilsons disease have normal ceruloplasmins.[6] Thus the practice of only obtaining a ceruloplasmin as reassurance that a young patient does not have Wilsons disease should be abandoned.

The Kayser–Fleischer ring is an accumulation of copper in Descemets membrane, and can be seen at the bedside by side illumination of the iris. However, definitive diagnosis requires a slit-lamp examination by an experienced ophthalmologist. This should be performed to secure the diagnosis, and also to obtain photographs of the rings to document clinical response to treatment. A Kayser–Fleischer ring is shown in Fig. 11.2. Neurologic Wilsons disease without documented Kayser–Fleischer rings is extremely rare.[7]

The major obstacle in the diagnosis of Wilsons disease is thinking of the disorder. Wilsons disease should be considered in the differential diagnosis of any patient who presents with a neurologic or psychiatric disorder, particularly in young patients who were previously well. Much of the difficulty in diagnosis results from the wide spectrum of presentations which bring the patient to medical attention. Neurologic presentations of Wilsons disease typically occur within the second decade, and are summarized in Table 11.1.[8] Wilson himself recognized tremor as a prominent clinical sign in his original description of the disorder.[4] Speech disturbance, sialorrhea, upper extremity tremor, and personality change are common early symptoms. Classic stigmata of parkinsonism,

Table 11.1. Neurologic presenting symptoms and signs of Wilsons disease.[8]

	Symptoms	Signs
Personality change	44 (32%)	27 (20%)
Speech	105 (77%)	53 (39%)
Sialorrhea	53 (39%)	29 (21%)
Dysphagia	21 (15%)	N/A
Open mouth	N/A	10 (7%)
Tongue abnormality	N/A	20 (15%)
Extraocular muscle abnormality	N/A	8 (6%)
Parkinsonian fascies	N/A	20 (15%)
Clumsy hand	52 (38%)	N/A
Bradykinesia	N/A	9 (7%)
Arm tremor	103 (76%)	40 (29%)
Arm dystonia	N/A	27 (20%)
Arm involuntary movement	N/A	8 (6%)
Leg tremor	N/A	8 (6%)
Leg dystonia	N/A	12 (9%)
Leg involuntary movement	N/A	2 (1%)
Gait	52 (38%)	13 (10%)

risor sardonicus, gaping mouth and limb dystonia are uncommon early in the disorder.

Denny-Brown and others differentiated between the 'pseudosclerotic' and 'progressive lenticular degeneration' presentations of Wilsons disease. As opposed to the lenticular form that presents early with dystonia, athetosis and cognitive disturbance, pseudosclerotic patients typically present with tremor in their late teens or early twenties, have little hepatic dysfunction and respond well to chelation therapy.[9] Pseudosclerotic patients usually have focal lesions in the thalamus, disrupting cerebello-thalamo-cortical connections.[10] Our patient's clinical profile fits best with this pseudosclerotic pattern. As discussed earlier, although certain features of his examination were reminiscent of essential tremor (vocal tremor and kinetic arm tremor), the frequency of his tremor and its proximal distribution were inconsistent with this diagnosis.

There is tremendous phenotypic variability both between patients with different mutations in the ATP7B gene, and even within families where several individuals share the same mutation.[1,11] Nevertheless, patients with the His1069Gln mutation often present, as our patient did, with neurologic symptoms late in their second decade.[1,11] The majority of Wilsons disease patients are heterozygous, carrying different mutations in their two gene alleles. Homozygous patients offer an opportunity to correlate a clinical phenotype with a specific gene mutation. Our patient's mutation was the most common mutation in these patients, present in 38% of patients in one series.[1] It is typically seen in North American, Swedish and Russian patients[1] (both of our patient's parents had Ukrainian ancestors).

Occasionally the diagnosis of Wilsons disease is suggested by the results of neuroimaging in a patient who presents with an unusual movement disorder. The MRI is usually abnormal in a Wilsons disease patient with neurologic symptoms and signs.[12] In addition to atrophy, high signal on T2 images is commonly seen in the basal ganglia, brainstem, thalamus and occasionally the white matter. Aside from involvement of the lateral thalamus, our patient's MRI displayed selective white matter tract abnormalities, including lesions in the corpus callosum. This pattern is occasionally seen in Wilsons disease. Internal capsule, cerebellar peduncle and even centrum semiovale can be abnormal, although corpus callosum abnormalities are distinctly unusual.[13]

The treatment of Wilsons disease has changed dramatically over the last four decades. Since the disorder is genetic, all family members who could be affected should be screened for the disorder. Foods high in copper (liver and shellfish) should be avoided. There is considerable debate regarding the appropriate choice of decoppering agent in Wilsons disease. Patients with neurologic symptoms of Wilsons disease are at risk for neurologic deterioration during treatment with copper chelators. This deterioration may be permanent and devastating, and has been reported during treatment with penicillamine, the most frequently prescribed medication for this condition.[14] An alternate approach has been suggested, using zinc, trientine or tetrathiomolybdate, although the last drug is available only through clinical trials.[14] Given the rarity of the disease and the complexity of treatment, it seems prudent for a newly diagnosed patient with Wilsons disease to be referred to a tertiary level center with expertise in the management of this disorder.

If Wilsons disease is diagnosed early, even patients with severe neurologic abnormalities may return to normal. Unfortunately, patients who present late in their course, or who evidence brain atrophy on MRI frequently do not fully recover. Our patient's history illustrates the difficulty and importance of early diagnosis of this treatable condition.

Diagnosis

Wilsons disease.

References

1. Elble RJ. The pathophysiology of tremor. In: Watts RL, Koller WC, eds. *Movement Disorders*. New York: McGraw-Hill, 1997: 405–417.
2. Koller WC, Busenbark KL. Essential tremor. In Watts RL, Koller WC, eds. *Movement Disorders*. New York: McGraw-Hill, 1997: 365–385.
3. Shah AB, Chernov I, Zhang HT et al. Identification and analysis of mutations in the Wilson disease gene (ATP7B): population frequencies, genotype–phenotype correlation, and functional analyses. *Am J Hum Genet* 1997; **61:** 317–328.

4. Wilson SAK. Progressive lenticular degeneration: a familial nervous disease associated with cirrhosis of the liver. *Brain* 1912; **34:** 295–509.
5. Saito T. Presenting symptoms and natural history of Wilson disease. *Eur J Pediatr* 1987; **146:** 261–265.
6. Brewer GJ, Fink JK, Hedera P. Diagnosis and treatment of Wilsons disease. *Semin Neurol* 1999; **19:** 261–270.
7. Ross E, Jacobson IM, Dienstag JL, Martin JB. Late onset Wilsons disease with neurologic involvement in the absence of Kayser–Fleischer rings. *Ann Neurol* 1985; **17:** 411–413.
8. Walshe JM, Yealland M. Wilsons disease: the problem of delayed diagnosis. *J Neurol Neurosurg Psychiatry* 1992; **55:** 692–696.
9. Denny-Brown D. Hepatolenticular degeneration (Wilsons disease). *New Engl J Med* 1964; **270:** 1149–1156.
10. Oder W, Prayer L, Grimm G et al. Wilsons disease: evidence of subgroups derived from clinical findings and brain lesions. *Neurology* 1993; **43:** 120–124.
11. Petrukhin K, Lutsenko S, Chernov I, Ross BM, Kaplan JH, Gilliam TC. Characterization of the Wilson disease gene encoding a P-type copper transporting ATPase: genomic organization, alternative splicing, and structure/function predictions. *Hum Mol Genet* 1994; **3:** 1647–1656.
12. Saatci I, Topcu M, Baltaoglu FF et al. Cranial MR findings in Wilsons disease. *Acta Radiologica* 1997; **38:** 250–258.
13. Van Wassenaer, van Hall HN, van den Heuvel AG, Algra A, Hoogenraad TU, Mali WPTM. Wilsons disease: findings at MR imaging and CT of the brain with clinical correlation. *Radiology* 1996; **198:** 531–536.
14. Brewer GJ. Penicillamine should not be used as initial therapy in Wilsons disease. *Mov Disord* 1999; **14:** 551–554.

12

Muscle weakness and dysphagia

Clinical history and examination

A 60-year-old carpenter presented with slowly progressive weakness of his legs.

The leg weakness had been of insidious onset, progressing over a period of approximately 10 years. He had a recent tendency to fall unexpectedly. He had noticed some loss of muscle bulk in his legs and arms. He had also experienced difficulty with fine tasks in the hands, including difficulty in holding nails, and using a hammer. On closer questioning, he had noticed occasional difficulty with swallowing for the past year, and had recent onset of dyspepsia.

Diabetes mellitus had been diagnosed 5 years previously, and this was treated with dietary control. He was taking antacids for dyspepsia, but no other medication. He had recently had gastrosopic examination, and been diagnosed as having an early gastric carcinoma. There was no other relevant medical history. There was no family history of neurologic disease.

His temperature was 37.0°C, pulse was 78, and respirations were 16 per minute. The blood pressure was 145/90 mmHg.

On physical examination, there was mild generalized muscle wasting, with marked wasting of the quadriceps femoris and forearm muscles. There was moderate weakness of knee extension bilaterally, and mild weakness of finger and wrist flexion bilaterally. Sensation was normal in the upper limbs. There was diminution of soft touch and pinprick sensation in the feet, with reduced vibration sensation in the toes, but normal proprioception. Tone and coordination were normal in the limbs. Deep tendon reflexes were absent at the ankles, diminished at the knees, and normal in the arms. Plantar responses were flexor bilaterally. When walking there was weakness at the knees, with some instability.

There was mild weakness of the facial muscles, but the remainder of the cranial nerve examination was normal.

The urine demonstrated a moderate amount of glucose. Hematologic laboratory findings included a mild anaemia elevated ESR (42 mm/h), and normal white cell count and platelet count. The blood film was microcytic. Blood chemical findings included a raised nonfasting glucose (10.5 mmol/l), normal sodium, potassium, and urea, normal liver enzymes, and normal thyroid function tests. Creatine kinase was mildly raised at 190 IU/l (normal < 100 IU/l). Serum ferritin and iron were reduced.

MRI of the lumbosacral spine demonstrated degenerative discs at L4/5 and L5/S1, but no impingement of the discs on the nerve roots.

Nerve conduction studies demonstrated absent sural sensory action potentials bilaterally, but upper limb sensory studies were within normal limits. Motor conduction velocities in the upper and lower limbs were normal. Electromyography of the right quadriceps femoris demonstrated moderate fibrillations and positive sharp waves at rest. There was rapid recruitment of low amplitude, short duration polyphasic potentials, with a mild reduction in interference pattern.

A diagnostic test was performed.

*   *   *

Discussion

This 60-year-old man presented with progressive weakness and wasting of quadriceps muscles, together with features of a sensory neuropathy.

The differential diagnosis includes a femoral neuropathy, radiculopathy, or plexopathy; a more generalized neuropathy, or a myopathy. He has diabetes mellitus, the most likely explanation of the sensory changes and absent ankle reflexes. However, a diabetic femoral neuropathy or radiculoplexopathy, causing diabetic amyotropy, should be considered. This condition is often associated with pain, which was not a feature in this patient. The ESR is moderately raised, and an inflammatory, or vasculitic, neuropathy should also be considered. Nerve conduction studies have not demonstrated any more widespread features of a mononeuritis multiplex to support this. Carcinomatous plexopathy is a consideration in a man of this age. Magnetic resonance imaging of the lumbosacral spine has excluded any structural, and surgically treatable, cause for the weakness and wasting of the quadriceps muscle.

The diminished, but preserved, knee reflexes, in the presence of significant weakness and wasting of the muscle, would suggest that this is not a primary neuropathic weakness. A proximal myopathy would cause similar features, and is supported by the EMG findings. The spontaneous activity at rest, with fibrillation potentials and positive sharp waves suggests an active inflammatory myositis.

There are three main forms of inflammatory myositis. These are polymyositis, dermatomyositis, and inclusion body myositis.[1]

Polymyositis usually presents in women. Initial symptoms are of weakness of proximal arms and legs, or neck flexion. Distal muscles may also be weak. There may be associated pain or tenderness of the muscles. Oropharyngeal and esophageal involvement may cause dysphagia. There may be a slight increased risk of associated malignancy.[2] Serum creatine kinase is usually significantly raised. The EMG findings are those found in other inflammatory myopathies, with increased insertional and spontaneous activity, and small amplitude short duration polyphasic units, with rapid recruitment. Muscle biopsy shows characteristic features, with variability in fiber size, necrotic and regenerating fibers, and endomysial inflammation including invasion of non-necrotic muscle fibers. Major histocompatibility complex (MHC) class I expression may be a useful indication of the inflammatory component. The inflammatory cells are predominantly CD8 positive T cells, with macrophages.[3,4] This reflects the antigen-specific, cell-mediated immune response pathogenesis of polymyositis. The primary antigen is not known. Most patients with polymyositis respond to treatment with immunosuppressive agents, which may initially include prednisone and azathioprine.[1,5]

Dermatomyositis may present in children or adults, and is relatively common in childhood, with some distinctive clinical features. Women are affected more commonly than men. In adults the presentation is usually with proximal limb, or neck flexion, weakness. In children the presentation may be with nonspecific features including fatigue, low grade fever, and rash, followed by muscle weakness and myalgia. Oropharyngeal and esophageal muscle involvement may cause dysphagia in around 30% of patients.

A distinctive feature of dermatomyositis is the rash, which may precede or follow the onset of muscle weakness. This typically includes a heliotrope rash (purplish discoloration of the eyelids), and Grottons sign (papular, erythematous, scaly lesions over the knuckles). A flat, erythematous, photosensitive rash may be present on the face, neck, chest, shoulders, upper back, elbows, knees, and ankles. Dilated capillary loops, with hemorrhage or thrombosis, may be present in the nail beds. Subcutaneous calcification is common in children with dermatomyositis (30–70%), but is rarer in adults. This may cause painful hard nodules which may ulcerate.[6] Cardiac arrhythmia and myocarditis may complicate dermatomyositis, and 10% of patients develop interstitial lung disease. Vasculitis may occur in the gastrointestinal tract, leading to ulceration and hemorrhage.

There is an increased risk of associated malignancy in adult dermatomyositis, although the extent of this is controversial. Published risks range from 6 to 45%.[1,2,7] Muscle strength may improve with treatment of the underlying malignancy. Careful enquiry for symptoms of malignancy, and thorough physical examination, should be performed. Investigation is usually limited to routine blood tests, fecal occult bloods, chest X-ray, and mammography, unless additional symptoms or signs indicate additional investigation.

Serum creatine kinase is usually significantly raised, although may be normal. Electromyography shows similar features to the other inflammatory myopathies (see above). Muscle biopsy shows distinctive features, in particular perifascicular atrophy, with degenerating fibers. Inflammatory infiltration of macrophages, B cells, and CD4 positive T cells, is predominantly perivascular, and in the perimysium rather than endomysium. There may be necrosis of small blood vessel walls, with deposition of a complement membrane attack complex. These features suggest that dermatomyositis is a humorally mediated microangiopathy, leading to ischemic damage of muscle fibers.[8,9] Hence, while the clinical definition of dermatomyositis suggests the importance of finding a skin rash, the distinctive pathogenetic features of the condition are demonstrated by muscle biopsy.

Treatment of dermatomyositis is usually with prednisone, and sometimes azathioprine.[1] Most patients respond to therapy, but associated malignancy may determine the overall prognosis.

The most common myopathy in patients over age 50 years is inclusion body myositis (IBM).[1,10,11] This has distinctive clinical features. It is most often a disease of middle aged or elderly men. It is more frequent in men, unlike polymyositis which is more common in women. Weakness usually starts in the lower limbs, especially quadriceps muscles. Weakness is also found in the forearm muscles, especially finger flexors and wrist flexors, more than extensors. The involvement of these muscle groups is especially suggestive of inclusion body myositis. Facial muscles may be involved, but extraocular muscles are spared. Dysphagia may develop in up to 40% of patients, and may be severe.[12] The limb weakness may be asymmetrical. The disease is slowly progressive. The distinctive morphological diagnostic feature is of rimmed vacuolar inclusions in muscle fibers.

Inclusion body myositis is a sporadic disease, but other myopathies may be associated with inclusion bodies. These are termed hereditary inclusion body myopathies (h-IBM). There is generally no inflammatory change, and hence the term myopathy rather than myositis for the hereditary forms. These include some of the distal myopathies:[13] Welander distal myopathy (found especially in Sweden),[14] Nonaka distal myopathy (found especially in Japan),[15] Markesbery–Griggs/Udd distal myopathy (found especially in Finland),[16,17] and the quadriceps sparing vacuolar myopathy of Persian Jews (or autosomal recessive hereditary inclusion body myopathy),[18] which has now been demonstrated to be genetically associated with Nonaka myopathy (Table 12.1).

Table 12.1. Distal myopathies, including vacuolar myopathies.

Type	Inheritance	Initial weakness	CK	Biopsy	Gene
Nonaka – early adult onset type I (familial IBM*)	Autosomal recessive or sporadic	Legs: anterior compartment	Slightly to moderately increased, usually < 5X	Vacuolar myopathy	9p1–q1
Miyoshi – early adult onset type II (LGMD 2B**)	Autosomal recessive or sporadic	Legs: posterior compartment	Increased 10–150X normal	Myopathic, usually without vacuoles; gastrocnemius often 'end stage'	2p13 dysferlin
Laing – early adult onset type III	Autosomal dominant	Legs: anterior compartment neck flexors	Slightly increased, < 3X normal	Moderate myopathic changes/no vacuoles	14q11
Welander – late adult type I	Autosomal dominant	Hands: fingers/wrist extensors	Normal or slightly increased	Myopathic; vacuoles in some cases	2p13
Markesbery – Griggs/Udd late adult onset type II	Autosomal dominant	Legs: anterior compartment	Normal or slightly increased	Vacuolar myopathy	2q31–33

* Autosomal recessive familial inclusion body myopathy (IBM), also known as quadriceps sparing myopathy, has been genetically linked with Nonaka distal myopathy.
** Limb girdle muscular dystrophy type 2B co-localizes with Miyoshi distal myopathy.

Further investigation and management

Biopsy of the left quadriceps femoris muscle (Fig. 12.1) demonstrated variation of fiber size, with occasional fibers up to 150 microns, and numerous small angular fibers and necrotic fibers. There were occasional foci of inflammatory change, and infiltrating cells were positive for CD8 T-lymphocyte markers. Vacuoles were present in many necrotic and non-necrotic fibers, some of the vacuoles being rimmed by basophilic material. Occasional (2%) ragged red fibers were present, with several SDH positive, COX negative, fibers. ATPase demonstrated atrophic fibers to be both Type I and Type II, with no grouping of fiber types. Staining for glycogen, lipid, and phosphorylase was normal. Further electron microscopic examination demonstrated cytoplasmic tubulofilaments, 16–21 nm diameter, in the vacuoles.

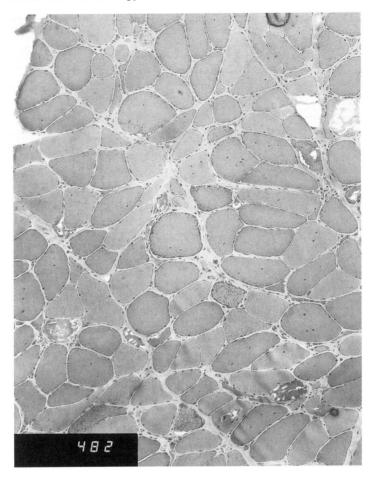

Fig. 12.1. Muscle biopsy stained with the modified Gomori trichrome stain. This demonstrates numerous fibers with rimmed vacuoles in addition to significant variation in fibers size with several small, often angulated fibres. There was only a minor degree of inflammatory change in this biopsy.

The muscle biopsy findings confirm the diagnosis of inclusion body myositis. The rimmed vacuoles may be infrequent, especially in the early stages of the disease, and an adequate specimen of muscle is important. Repeat biopsy after an interval may be indicated if the clinical suspicion is high and the first biopsy is not diagnostic. Vacuoles may be found in necrotic fibers as a nonspecific finding in muscle disease, and it is the finding of rimmed vacuoles in non-necrotic muscle fibers which is distinctive. Amyloid may be demonstrated in non-necrotic vacuolated muscle fibers using fluorescent Congo Red staining.[19,20] The vacuolated muscle fibers contain cytoplasmic tubulofilaments, with diameters of 16–21 nm.[12] Similar tubulofilaments are present in the nucleus. Ragged red fibers may also be found in the muscle of patients with IBM.[21] Mitochondrial DNA mutations are also more frequent in patients with IBM,[22] but these are thought to be secondary changes, and not a primary cause of the disease.

The pathogenesis of IBM is unknown. The endomysial inflammation comprises macrophages and CD8 positive T lymphocytes invading non-necrotic muscle fibers. These features are similar to polymyositis. However, in contra-distinction to polymyositis, the T-cell response in IBM appears not to be directed against a muscle specific antigen.[23,24] Although this may be a primary inflammatory myopathy (as are derma-tomyositis and polymyositis), a primary degenerative myopathy has also been considered. For example, proteins found in Alzheimers disease have been found in IBM inclusions. These include B-amyloid, B-amyloid precursor protein, prion protein, apolipoprotein E, α1-antichymotrypsin, ubiquitin, hyperphosphorylated tau protein, and neurofilament heavy chain.[10,25]

At present there is no treatment with demonstrated efficacy for inclusion body myositis. Immunosuppressive treatments including prednisone and azathioprine, and intravenous immunoglobulin infusion, which have efficacy in dermatomyositis and polymyositis, do not alter the course of IBM.[1,26]

Diagnosis

Inclusion body myositis.

References

1. Amato AA, Barohn RJ. Inflammatory myopathies: dermatomyositis, polymyo-sitis, inclusion body myositis, and related diseases. In: Schapira AHV, Griggs RC, eds. Muscle Diseases. Boston: Butterworth-Heinemann, 1999; 299–338.
2. Sigurgeirsson B, Lindelof B, Edhag O et al. Risk of cancer in patient with dermatomyositis or polymyositis. N Engl J Med 1992; 326: 363–367.
3. Arahata K, Engel AG. Monoclonal antibody analysis of mononuclear cells in myopathies. I: Quantitative subsets according to diagnosis and sites of accu-mulation and demonstration and counts of muscle fibers invaded by T cells. Ann Neurol 1984; 16: 193–208.
4. Engel AG, Arahata K. Monoclonal antibody analysis of mononuclear cells in myopathies. II: Phenotypes of autoinvasive cells in polymyositis and inclusion body myositis. Ann Neurol 1984; 16: 209–215.
5. Joffe MM, Love LA, Leff RL. Drug therapy of idiopathic inflammatory myopathies: predictors of response to prednisone, azathioprine, and methotrex-ate and a comparison of their efficacy. Am J Med 1993; 94: 379–387.
6. Orrell RW, Johnston HM, Gibson C, Cass RM, Griggs RC. Spontaneous abdominal hematoma in dermatomyositis. Muscle Nerve 1998; 21: 1800–1803.
7. Callen JP. Relationship of cancer to inflammatory muscle diseases: dermato-myositis, polymyositis and dermatomyositis. Rheum Dis Clin North Am 1994; 20: 943–953.

8. Emslie-Smith AM, Engel AG. Microvascular changes in early and advanced dermatomyositis: a quantitative study. *Ann Neurol* 1990; **27:** 343–356.
9. Kissel JT, Halterman RK, Rammohan KW, Mendell JR. The relationship of complement-mediated microvasculopathy to the histologic features and clinical duration of disease in dermatomyositis. *Arch Neurol* 1991; **48:** 26–30.
10. Griggs RC, Askanas V, DiMauro S et al. Inclusion body myositis and myopathies. *Ann Neurol* 1995; **38:** 705–713.
11. Askanas V, Serratrice G, Engel WK, eds. *Inclusion-body Myositis and Myopathies.* Cambridge: Cambridge University Press, 1998.
12. Lotz BP, Engel AG, Nishino H et al. Inclusion body myositis. Observations in 40 patients. *Brain* 1989; **112:** 727–747.
13. Orrell RW, Griggs RC. Muscular dystrophies: overview of clinical and molecular approaches. In: Schapira AHV, Griggs RC, eds. *Muscle Diseases.* Boston: Butterworth-Heinemann, 1999: 59–82.
14. Welander L. Myopathia distalis tarda hereditaria. *Acta Med Scand* 1951; **141** (suppl. 265): 1–124.
15. Nonaka I, Sunohara N, Ihiura S, Satoyoshi E. Familial distal myopathy with rimmed vacuole and lamellar (myeloid) body formation. *J Neurol Sci* 1981; **51:** 141–155.
16. Markesbery WR, Griggs RC, Leach RP, Lapham LW. Late onset hereditary distal myopathy. *Neurology* 1974; **23:** 127–134.
17. Udd B, Partanen J, Halonen P et al. Tibial muscular dystrophy. Late adult-onset distal myopathy in 66 Finnish patients. *Arch Neurol* 1993; **50:** 604–608.
18. Mitrani-Rosenbaum S, Argov Z, Blumenfeld A et al. Hereditary inclusion body myopathy maps to chromosome 9p1-q1. *Hum Mol Genet* 1996; **5:** 159–163.
19. Mendell JR, Sahenk Z, Gales T et al. Amyloid filaments in inclusion body myositis. Novel findings provide insight into nature of filaments. *Arch Neurol* 1991; **48:** 1229–1234.
20. Askanas V, Engel WK, Alvarez RB. Enhanced detection of amyloid deposits in muscle fibers of inclusion body myositis and brain of Alzheimer's disease using fluorescence technique. *Neurology* 1993; **43:** 1265–1267.
21. Rifai Z, Welle S, Kamp C, Thornton CA. Ragged red fibers in normal aging and inflammatory myopathy. *Ann Neurol* 1995; **37:** 24–25.
22. Oldfors A, Larsson NG, Lindberg C et al. Mitochondrial DNA deletions in inclusion body myositis. *Brain* 1993; **116:** 325–336.
23. Mantegazza R, Andreetta F, Bernasconi P et al. Analysis of T cell receptor repertoire of muscle-infiltrating T lymphocytes in polymyositis. Restricted Valpha/beta rearrangements may indicate antigen-driven selection. *J Clin Invest* 1993; **91:** 2880–2886.
24. O'Hanlon TP, Dalakas MC, Plotz PH et al. The alpha-beta T-cell receptor repertoire in inclusion body myositis: diverse patterns of gene expression by infiltrating lymphocytes. *J Autoimmun* 1994; **7:** 321–333.
25. Askanas V, Engel WK, Bilak M et al. Twisted tubulofilaments of inclusion body myositis resemble paired helical filaments of Alzheimer brain and contain hyperphosphorylated tau. *Am J Pathol* 1994; **144:** 177–187.
26. Barohn RJ, Amato AA, Sahenk Z et al. Inclusion body myositis: explanation for poor response to therapy. *Neurology* 1995; **45:** 1302–1304.

13

Locked in?

Clinical history and examination

A 75-year-old woman was admitted to the hospital because of a change in mental status.

She was active and in good health until 2 days before admission, when she complained of not feeling well. Her son said that she appeared excessively tired. Over the next 24 hours, she became less communicative and spent most of the day in bed. With her son's help, she was able to take her medications and a small amount of food. On the evening before admission, she had a generalized convulsive seizure, which lasted less than 2 minutes. Following the seizure, she slept, snoring heavily. When her son tried to awaken her the next morning, he found her staring blankly, unresponsive to voice or touch. He called the paramedics for emergency assistance.

The patient had had hypertension and hypothyroidism for many years, and Parkinsons disease had been diagnosed 10 years before. She had a history of epilepsy 'many years ago,' and although the son was unaware of any details, he reported that she had not had a seizure in more than 5 years.

The patient's recent medications included phenytoin, carbidopa–levodopa, levothyroxine, atenolol, and multivitamins.

There was no history of recent fever, rash, cardiac or gastrointestinal symptoms, or head trauma. There was also no history of alcohol or drug use, or of psychiatric illness.

Physical examination in the emergency room revealed a rectal temperature of 98.6°F, pulse rate of 96, and respiratory rate of 16. The blood pressure was 130/80 mmHg. She was lying supine, without obvious movement, but did not appear ill. There was no rash or lymphadenopathy. There were no signs of head trauma. Kernig and Brudzinski signs were absent. There were no bruits. Breath sounds were clear. The heart rate and sounds were normal; there were no murmurs. The abdomen was soft and non-tender. There was no edema or cyanosis of the limbs.

Table 13.1. Blood chemical values.

Sodium (mmol/l)	138
Potassium (mmol/l)	3.9
Chloride (mmol/l)	101
Carbon dioxide (mmol/l)	24
Blood urea nitrogen (mg/dl)	13
Creatinine (mg/dl)	0.6
Glucose (mg/dl)	93
Calcium (mg/dl)	9.2
Magnesium (mEq/l)	1.9
Phosphate (mg/dl)	3.9
Creatine kinase (U/l)	45
Albumin (g/dl)	3.9
Alkaline phosphatase (U/l)	105
Alanine aminotransferase (U/l)	19
Aspartate aminotransferase (U/l)	21
Total bilirubin (mg/dl)	0.6
Ammonia (μmol/l)	29
Thyroid-stimulating hormone (μU/ml)	0.7
Thyroxine, total (μg/dl)	7.9
Phenytoin (mg/dl)	5.0

On neurological examination, the patient was lying supine without spontaneous limb or eye movements. Her eyes were open and fixed in primary gaze. There were occasional, small amplitude repetitive movements of the left eyebrow, which lasted 1–2 seconds. She did not respond to her name or other verbal stimuli. She groaned in response to a firm sternal rub and moved her arms and legs minimally in response to other noxious stimuli. There were no purposeful movements. Fundi were normal, and both pupils were 4 mm, round, and briskly reactive to light. There was no blink to threat. The oculocephalic reflex demonstrated full, conjugate eye movements. Corneal reflexes were symmetric. Facial appearance was symmetric, as was her grimace in response to pressure on the supraorbital nerve. Her gag reflex was weak but present, and her tongue and uvula were midline. Tone was mildly increased in the neck, arms and legs. There was no tremor or other adventitious movements. Deep tendon reflexes were 1+ throughout except at the ankles, where they were absent. Plantar responses were silent (neither flexor nor extensor).

Initial laboratory test results are shown in Tables 13.1 and 13.2. Thyroid function tests, done 1 month before admission, are also included in Table 13.1. The results of a lumbar puncture are shown in Table 13.3. Electrocardiogram, chest X-ray, and urinalysis were normal. Urine screen for toxins was negative. A specimen of arterial blood, drawn while the patient was breathing room air, showed a pO_2 of 86 mmHg, pCO_2 of 41 mmHg, and pH of 7.39. A computed tomographic (CT) head scan,

Table 13.2. Hematologic laboratory values.

Hematocrit	40%
Mean corpuscular volume	$91\,\mu m^3$
White cell count	$7.4\,per\,mm^3$
Differential count (%)	
Neutrophils	56%
Lymphocytes	35%
Monocytes	8%
Eosinophils	1%
Platelet count	$381\,per\,mm^3$
Prothrombin time	13.1 s
Partial thromboplastin time	23.2 s

Table 13.3. Results of lumbar puncture.

Opening pressure (mmH_2O)	140
Appearance of fluid	clear, colorless
White cells (per mm^3)	1
Red cells (per mm^3)	48
Glucose (mg/dl)	60
Protein (mg/dl)	19
Stained smear	no microorganisms

obtained without intravenous injection of contrast material, showed mild cerebral atrophy and small, bilateral frontal subdural hygromas, which were judged to be clinically insignificant. There were no infarctions, hemorrhages, or mass lesions.

A diagnostic procedure was performed.

*   *   *

Discussion

In approaching this case, it is useful first to identify the most important clinical features. This elderly woman with Parkinsons disease, epilepsy, and hypothyroidism had a gradual deterioration in her mental status over 2 days. Several hours after a brief, generalized convulsion, she was found unresponsive. Her examination revealed unresponsiveness and intermittent twitching of the left eyebrow but little else. In particular, there were no lateralizing findings or indications of brainstem dysfunction.

Loss of consciousness with preserved brainstem reflexes results from diffuse, bilateral depression of cerebral hemispheric function. The absence of significant focal findings virtually eliminates an underlying mass lesion clinically, and this was confirmed by CT head scan. The normal laboratory studies also exclude common causes of toxic-metabolic encephalopathy such as hypoxemia, hypercarbia, hypo/hyperglycemia, hypo/hypernatremia, hypo/hyperosmolality, hypo/hypercalcemia, uremia, and hyperammonemia. Depressant drugs are unlikely clinically because respiratory function was not compromised, and her pupils and eye movements were normal. Urine toxicology confirmed absence of opiates, barbiturates, and benzodiazepines.

While the patient was not hypoxic at the time of examination in the emergency ward, it is possible that she may have had an hypoxic brain injury during the night, especially if she had had several prolonged generalized convulsive seizures. This scenario is unlikely, however, given the normal serum creatine kinase. Convulsions severe enough to cause hypoxic encephalopathy are associated with muscle breakdown and elevation in creatine kinase. Furthermore, there was no ECG abnormality to suggest a primary cardiac event.

Central nervous system infection should always be considered in patients with altered consciousness. There were no signs to suggest meningitis or sepsis, and her cerebrospinal fluid (CSF) was normal. Viral encephalitis may present with mental status changes unaccompanied by fever and stiff neck, especially in elderly and immunocompromised individuals. Herpes simplex encephalitis, the most common cause of sporadic encephalitis in the USA, typically causes an acute or subacute alteration in mentation and behavior, seizures, and eventual coma. The spinal fluid is usually abnormal but may be normal in up to 10% of cases.[1] Subarachnoid hemorrhage is excluded by the normal CT and CSF.

The patient's medical history requires consideration of other possibilities. Chronic hypothyroidism can result in cognitive changes and, in its most severe form, 'myxedema coma.' In this elderly lady, the illness evolved too rapidly, and laboratory testing documented a euthyroid state in the recent past. Hashimotos encephalopathy, an immune-mediated disorder associated with high circulating levels of anti-thyroid antibodies, can lead to seizures, myoclonus, and coma. It is most common in euthyroid women.[2,3] Hashimotos encephalopathy is unlikely to be the cause of this woman's illness because its course is almost always more prolonged, and relapses and remissions are the rule. Furthermore, chronic cognitive and behavioral changes are prominent, and during exacerbations, there may be frequent seizures and transient focal neurological deficits suggesting small strokes. Cerebrospinal fluid protein is elevated in the majority of cases.

Because of the history of Parkinsons disease, the possibility of neuroleptic malignant syndrome (NMS), which can occur during withdrawal of dopaminergic therapy,[4,5] must be considered. Although patients with NMS have gradual deterioration in consciousness over a few days and often lapse into coma, fever, severe muscle rigidity and autonomic instability are invariable findings.

One of the most important findings in this patient was that her eyes were open. True coma manifests as unresponsiveness with eyes closed.[6] Lack of responsiveness with eyes open shifts the diagnostic focus to conditions that mimic coma. Patients who appear unresponsive but whose eyes are open may be 'locked-in,' a term introduced in 1966 by Plum and Posner.[6] They described patients with quadriplegia, paralysis of the lower cranial nerves, preserved vertical gaze and movement of the upper eyelids, and no alteration in consciousness. The inability to respond, resulting in apparent 'coma' with eyes open, results from de-efferentation caused by large destructive lesions of the basis pontis which spare the ascending reticular activating system and vertical gaze centers in the midbrain. Since the original description, variations in presentation have been described, and Bauer et al.[7] have proposed classifying patients with the locked-in syndrome into three groups: (1) classical cases as described by Plum and Posner; (2) incomplete cases in whom various motor functions other than vertical gaze and blinking are preserved to some extent; and (3) cases with complete paralysis – no movement in any muscle – but EEGs demonstrating normal wake and sleep patterns. In a large series of 139 cases, Patterson and Grabois[8] classified 46 patients as examples of 'incomplete' locked-in syndrome. Nearly one-third of these had preservation of some motor response in the extremities, and more than half had partial preservation of horizontal eye movements. In addition, the majority of patients had premonitory symptoms, including generalized weakness and alteration in mental status, usually during the preceding 24 hours.[8] The possibility of an atypical locked-in syndrome is excluded in this patient by the findings on neurological examination. The patient made no attempt to communicate by blinking or eye movements; her extraocular movements were full to reflex testing; corneal and gag reflexes were intact; and facial and limb movements, although limited, were symmetric.

The two most likely diagnoses are catatonia and non-convulsive status epilepticus. Catatonic patients often appear to be in a coma-like state. Catatonia is a psychiatric syndrome in which motor anomalies and other disturbances in motor function result from functional or psychological disorders rather than from neurological conditions that are demonstrably due to physiological, biochemical, or anatomic abnormalities affecting the brain.[9] When motor activity slows to the point of immobility and there is apparent inability to communicate with loss of awareness of surroundings, the patient is said to be in a 'catatonic stupor.' The absence of a psychiatric history in this patient does not exclude catatonia. Several studies have found that only a minority of patients have a history of schizophrenia, and many suffer from affective disorder or have a history of neurological or medical illness.[10] Thus, the history of hypothyroidism and Parkinsons disease, both of which are associated with depression, might be construed as support for a diagnosis of catatonia. Furthermore, chronic treatment with levodopa may induce psychotic symptoms. More significant, however, is the lack of the single most characteristic feature of catatonic stupor: catalepsy. Catalepsy is especially prominent when severe catatonia produces a coma-like state. Nonetheless, it is difficult to exclude this diagnosis solely on clinical grounds, although the absence of catalepsy makes catatonia unlikely. It must be remembered that catatonia and non-convulsive status epilepticus can be quite difficult to distinguish by clinical examination alone. There are multiple case reports of 'ictal catatonia,' as well as reports of patients with catatonia mimicking non-convulsive status epilepticus.[11,12] Moreover, both disorders will show some degree of response to intravenous benzodiazepines.[10] Definitive distinction between the two conditions requires an EEG. In catatonia, the EEG is usually normal, although there may be excessive nonspecific slowing due to medications the patient has received. In any event, the EEG in catatonic stupor always demonstrates a striking disparity to the clinical state.

Non-convulsive status epilepticus (NCSE) refers to a state characterized by persistent slowness in behavior and mentation, confusion, and sometimes stupor or coma, accompanied by continuous electrographic ictal patterns.[13] Several aspects of this patient's presentation favor a diagnosis of NCSE. First, the picture of unresponsiveness with staring is consistent with epilepsy. Both absence and complex partial seizures, although much briefer events, share these features to some degree. Second, although manifestations of NCSE can be very heterogeneous, this patient illustrates a well-recognized form of presentation.[14] In one series, 25% of patients with NCSE were unresponsive to verbal stimuli.[14] Third, the intermittent left eyebrow twitching should suggest an underlying epileptic disorder. Indeed, Tomson and co-workers[14] found that the most frequent motor manifestation, occurring in more than 50% of their patients, was irregular, discrete muscle twitches of the eyelids, perioral region, or limbs. Fourth, the single generalized seizure and history of epilepsy make the diagnosis of NCSE more likely: a generalized tonic–clonic seizure may be the initial or an early feature in one-third to one-half of patients with NCSE.[14,15] Low antiepileptic drug (AED) levels, as found in this patient, have been associated with NCSE.[14,15] and may allow the emergence of the syndrome. Fifth, the evolution of this patient's illness, from altered mental state to semi-coma in 2 days, is typical. NCSE often has a subacute course, and it tends to fluctuate in severity. It may be days before it is recognized and a diagnosis made.[16] Finally, as is usual in NCSE,[17] the diagnostic evaluation was normal or non-contributory.

The diagnostic procedure was an electroencephalogram (EEG). This showed continuous, generalized, atypical sharp and slow wave discharges that recurred at a frequency of about 2 Hz (Fig. 13.1). Vigorous verbal and painful stimulation during the recording did not produce appreciable clinical or electrographic changes consistent with ongoing ictal activity.

The patient was given intravenous lorazepam, 2 mg, and loaded with

intravenous fosphenytoin, 15 mg/kg. Over the next 15 minutes, the generalized epileptiform discharges became less frequent and subsided completely
by 30 minutes. Post-ictal EEG activity was characterized by moderate
diffuse slow wave activity (Fig. 13.2). Re-examination demonstrated a
corresponding improvement in the patient's condition. She lay quietly in
bed with her eyes closed. Although lethargic, she opened her eyes to voice,
followed simple commands, and moved her arms and legs spontaneously.
The left eyebrow no longer twitched. One hour after injection, she was
asleep but aroused quickly to voice. She was oriented to person and year,
followed two-step commands, and spoke in brief, coherent sentences.
Except for signs of mild Parkinsons disease, the remainder of her neurological examination was normal. The following morning, her mental status
examination had returned to normal.

While several features of this patient's presentation suggested NCSE,
this entity is often a problematic diagnosis. Much of the difficulty in
diagnosis stems from the variability in clinical presentation. Although
patients may present in stupor or a coma-like state, this represents a
minority of cases.[17] More commonly, patients are alert but confused
with prominent behavioral changes ranging from apathy to bizarre
behavior.[14-16,18] Symptoms have usually been present for several hours
or days, sometimes even for weeks, and typically have a fluctuating or,
occasionally, progressive course.[14-16] Overt signs of seizure, such as tonic
postures, clonic movements, or myoclonic jerks, are infrequent.[14]
Consequently, the syndrome may mimic disorders other than epilepsy,
including dementia, psychosis, depression, encephalopathy, and stroke.

In addition to the variability in clinical presentation, diagnostic difficulty
also results from the absence of any history of epilepsy. As many as one-
third of patients with NCSE have not had previous seizures.[15] In a group
of critically ill elderly patients with NCSE, fewer than 10% had a history
of epilepsy.[19]

As a result, diagnosis of NCSE is frequently missed or delayed. In one
case series, a correct diagnosis was not made in nearly half the patients
until more than 24 hours after admission in nearly half the patients.[15] A
high index of suspicion, prompt EEG recording, and response to AED
treatment are criteria for diagnosis. NCSE cannot be diagnosed by
response to medication alone. Catatonia, especially, may improve rapidly
following intravenous benzodiazepines.[10] EEG is necessary both for
diagnosis and guiding treatment.

Accurate interpretation of EEG abnormalities is also essential, and an
appropriate electrographic–clinical correlation is required. Triphasic
waves, which are seen most often in the setting of metabolic encephalopathy, do not represent electrographic seizure activity.[20] Although
triphasic waves may attenuate after administration of benzodiazepines,
there is no associated clinical improvement.[20] In contrast, the EEG in
NCSE demonstrates continuous ictal activity. The usual finding, as in
this patient, is continuous, or nearly continuous, generalized, rhythmic,

0:11:30:13.00 15 sec 15 uV 1x 1 - BP1-lrlr 0.1 sec 70 Hz 60 Hz

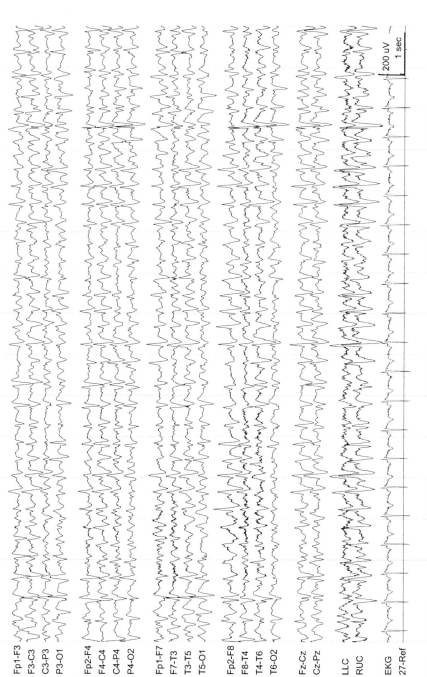

Fp1-F3				
F3-C3				
C3-P3				
P3-O1				

| Fp2-F4 |
| F4-C4 |
| C4-P4 |
| P4-O2 |

| Fp1-F7 |
| F7-T3 |
| T3-T5 |
| T5-O1 |

| Fp2-F8 |
| F8-T4 |
| T4-T6 |
| T6-O2 |

| Fz-Cz |
| Cz-Pz |

| LLC |
| RUC |

| EKG |
| 27-Ref |

200 uV
1 sec

Time 0:11:30:13   0:11:30:16   0:11:30:19   0:11:30:22   0:11:30:25

Fig. 13.1. Electroencephalogram obtained before treatment.

0:12:08:06.00 15 sec 15 uV 1x 1 - BP1-inr 0.1 sec 70 Hz 60 Hz

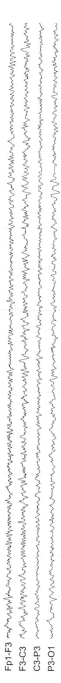

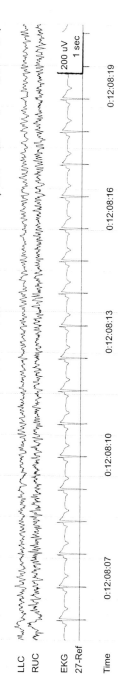

200 uV
1 sec

Time	0:12:08:07	0:12:08:10	0:12:08:13

0:12:08:16   0:12:08:19

Fig. 13.2. Electroencephalogram performed 30 minutes after injection of lorazepam intravenously.

1–2.5 Hz spike wave discharges.[13,17] In a minority of cases, the ictal discharges are localized, often to the frontal or temporal region of one hemisphere, thus indicating complex partial status epilepticus.[13,17] While it was once taught that complex partial status epilepticus typically manifested with fluctuations in behavior and level of consciousness, and that generalized NCSE presented with a more continuous pattern of change in mental status, it is now recognized that clinical semiology does not permit distinction between focal and generalized types of NCSE.[14,15] Two other observations have further blurred this difference: First, patients with a history of localization-related epilepsy who develop NCSE may show apparently generalized spike wave discharges, suggesting that such patterns may be *secondarily generalized*.[13,15] Second, there does not appear to be a differential response to AEDs between the two groups.[14]

Initial treatment is with intravenous benzodiazepines, usually lorazepam or diazepam. The clinical response may be either immediate or delayed. Tomson and colleagues[14] reported immediate improvement in almost all cases but noted that many patients required addition of phenytoin to achieve sustained benefit. In contrast, Kaplan[15] found that almost half the patients responded only after 24 hours of treatment. Seizures may recur in more than 60% of patients.[14] Thus, chronic AED therapy should be started after initial treatment with benzodiazepines. Continuous EEG monitoring, if available, is helpful until patients are stabilized. As with cases of convulsive status epilepticus, it is necessary to look for an underlying precipitant, such as metabolic derangement or unrecognized cerebral pathology. Often, however, no abnormality will be found.[17]

Unlike convulsive status epilepticus, the evidence for permanent neurological damage from NCSE is ambiguous. Experimental models have demonstrated neuronal injury from NCSE, but there is considerable controversy about lasting neurological dysfunction from NCSE in humans.[21,22] One complicating factor is that assessment of neurological outcome in NCSE is often confounded by comorbidity, especially in the elderly.[19] Furthermore, as mentioned previously, NCSE is a heterogeneous syndrome. Thus, attempts to assess outcome without differentiating patient populations have not provided meaningful results.[23]

NCSE is uncommon, although it is probably underrecognized. In a recent study of 236 consecutive comatose patients who had no clinical evidence of seizures, 8% had EEG findings consistent with NCSE.[24] In the same center, NCSE represented 5% of cases of status epilepticus.[24] Such data indicate that NCSE is not as rare as previously thought. With its varied clinical presentations, often mimicking other disorders, a high degree of suspicion for NCSE needs to be maintained in order to assure proper diagnosis and treatment.

Diagnosis

Non-convulsive status epilepticus.

References

1. Schlageter N, Burk J, Vick NA. Herpes simplex encephalitis without CSF leukocytosis. *Archives of Neurology* 1984; **41**: 1007–1008.
2. Kothbauer-Margreiter I, Sturzenegger M, Komor J et al. Encephalopathy associated with Hashimoto thyroiditis: diagnosis and treatment. *J Neurol* 1996; **243**: 585–593.
3. Shaw PJ, Walls TJ, Newman PK et al. Hashimoto's encephalopathy: a steroid-responsive disorder with high anti-thyroid antibody titers – report of 5 cases. *Neurology* 1991; **41**: 228–233.
4. Guze BH, Baxter LR Jr. Neuroleptic malignant syndrome. *N Engl J Med* 1985; **313**: 163–166.
5. Kornhuber J, Weller M. Neuroleptic malignant syndrome. *Curr Opin Neurol* 1994; **7**: 353–357.
6. Plum F, Posner JB. The Diagnosis of Stupor and Coma, 3rd edn. Philadelphia: FA Davis, 1983.
7. Bauer G, Gerstenbrand F, Rumpl E. Varieties of the locked-in syndrome. *J Neurol* 1979; **221**: 77–91.
8. Patterson JR, Grabois M. Locked-in syndrome: a review of 139 cases. *Stroke* 1986; **17**: 758–765.
9. American Psychiatric Association. *Diagnostic and Statistical Manual of Mental Disorders*, 4th edn. Washington, DC: American Psychiatric Association, 1994: 273–315.
10. Salam SA, Kilzieh N. Lorazepam treatment of psychogenic catatonia: an update. *J Clin Psychiat* 1988; **49** (12, suppl.): 16–21.
11. Lim JH, Yagnik P, Schraeder P et al. Ictal catatonia as a manifestation of nonconvulsive status epilepticus. *J Neurol Neurosurg Psychiatry* 1986; **49**: 833–836.
12. Louis ED, Pflaster NL. Catatonia mimicking nonconvulsive status epilepticus. *Epilepsia* 1995; **36**: 943–945.
13. Granner MA, Lee SI. Nonconvulsive status epilepticus: EEG analysis in a large series. *Epilepsia* 1994; **35**: 42–47.
14. Tomson T, Lindbom U, Nilsson BY. Nonconvulsive status epilepticus in adults: thirty-two consecutive patients from a general hospital population. *Epilepsia* 1992; **33**: 829–835.
15. Kaplan PW. Nonconvulsive status epilepticus in the emergency room. *Epilepsia* 1996; **37**: 643–650.
16. Scholtes FB, Renier WO, Meinardi H. Non-convulsive status epilepticus: causes, treatment, and outcome in 65 patients. *J Neurol Neurosurg Psychiatry* 1996; **61**: 93–95.
17. Pedley TA, Bazil CW, Morrell MJ. Epilepsy. In: Rowland LP, ed. *Merritt's Textbook of Neurology*, 10th edn. Baltimore: Lippincott, Williams and Wilkins, 2000; 813–833.
18. Williamson PD. Complex partial status epilepticus. In: Engel J, Pedley TA, eds. *Epilepsy: A Comprehensive Textbook*. Philadelphia: Lippincott-Raven, 1997.

19. Litt B, Wityk RJ, Hertz SH et al. Nonconvulsive status epilepticus in the critically ill elderly. *Epilepsia* 1998; **39:** 1194–1201.
20. Chatrian GE. Coma, other states of altered responsiveness, and brain death. In: Daly D, Pedley TA, eds. *Current Practice of Clinical Electroencephalography*, 2nd edn. Philadelphia: Lippincott-Raven Publishers, 1991; 425–487.
21. Drislane F. Evidence against permanent neurologic damage from nonconvulsive status epilepticus. *J Clin Neurophysiol* 1999; **16:** 323–331.
22. Krumholz A. Epidemiology and evidence for morbidity of nonconvulsive status epilepticus. *J Clin Neurophysiol* 1999; **16:** 314–322.
23. Kaplan PW. Assessing the outcomes in patients with nonconvulsive status epilepticus: nonconvulsive status epilepticus is underdiagnosed, potentially overtreated, and confounded by comorbidity. *J Clin Neurophysiol* 1999; **16:** 341–352.
24. Towne AR, Waterhouse EJ, Boggs JG et al. Prevalence of nonconvulsive status epilepticus in comatose patients. *Neurology* 2000; **54:** 340–345.

14

Optic neuritis and intracerebral mass

Clinical history and examination

This 42-year-old right-handed man awoke one night 8 months earlier with a severe right-sided retro-orbital headache associated with nausea. The headache was severe enough that he sought assistance in a local emergency room. A cranial CT, and subsequently MRI scan, revealed a right temporoparietal-enhancing lesion with mass effect and edema (Fig. 14.1). Chest X-ray and routine blood investigations were normal. The patient's past medical history was significant for right optic neuritis 6 years previously. He had no history of antecedent viral infections, vaccinations, insect bites, rashes, or fever. He had no family history of any neurologic illnesses. He did not use tobacco or illicit drugs but did occasionally drink alcohol. He had no occupational exposures or recent travel. He had two dogs. He denied risk factors for HIV.

On initial evaluation, his mental status examination was normal except for poor memory and concentration. He had a right afferent pupillary defect and a left facial droop. His tone was increased on the left and he had a left hemiparesis with greater weakness distally. He had hemianesthesia on the left to all sensory modalities but sparing his face. He had a broad-based stance and could only take small shuffling steps. He had 3+ deep tendon reflexes on the left, a left Babinski and Hoffmans sign. A diagnostic procedure was performed.

* * *

Discussion

This 42-year-old man had an acute right-sided headache and was found to have a right temporoparietal ring-enhancing lesion on MRI. The differential diagnosis of an enhancing intracranial mass is extensive.

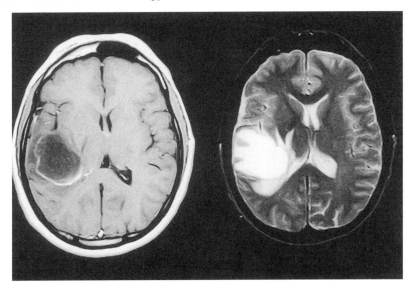

Fig. 14.1. Magnetic resonance imaging at presentation shows a cystic appearing lesion with an incomplete enhancing ring and associated edema. Left image is a contrast enhanced T1, and a T2 image is on the right.

The first consideration is a neoplasm, either a primary brain tumor or a metastasis. Approximately 20% of patients with systemic cancer present with brain metastases. In most patients, however, brain metastases occur late in their illness and after the diagnosis of cancer has been made. The most common symptoms of brain metastasis are headache and mental status change but seizures or focal neurologic deficits are often present. The most common tumors to metastasize to the brain are lung, breast and melanoma. On MRI, metastases are usually hypointense on T1 and hyperintense on T2. They are usually ring enhancing after contrast administration but can appear solid, cystic or mixed. They are well circumscribed, single in 25–50% of patients and tend to occur at the gray–white matter junction. Metastases from lung, melanoma, renal or thyroid primaries may have a hemorrhagic component. The absence of a smoking history and constitutional symptoms such as weight loss or fatigue, as well as the patient's normal general examination argue against the diagnosis of a metastatic tumor.

Primary brain tumors are usually derived from glia and occur at any age. Radiographically most low-grade tumors can be distinguished from high-grade tumors. Low-grade gliomas are usually non-enhancing infiltrative lesions with minimal mass effect and no edema. They are isointense to hypointense on T1 and homogeneously hyperintense on T2. Calcification can sometimes be seen, particularly in oligodendrogliomas. High-grade tumors are poorly delineated with mixed signal intensity on T1 (isointense to hypointense) and hyperintense on T2. There may be evidence of hemorrhage and necrosis; some lesions may have a cystic component. Contrast enhancement is irregular and ring-like. There is associated edema with varying mass effect. Both low- and high-grade lesions spread along white matter tracts and can involve the contralateral hemisphere. Low-grade gliomas can degenerate into higher grade tumors, usually years after the initial diagnosis. Low-grade gliomas often present with seizures and have a median age of onset in the third to fourth decade. Malignant astrocytomas have a medium age of onset in the fourth to sixth decade, and these patients usually present with seizures, headaches, confusion, or focal deficits. This patient's acute symptoms and the significant contrast enhancement of a large single lesion on MRI scan are consistent with a high-grade glial neoplasm, such as a glioblastoma multiforme.

Another primary brain tumor that can present with symptoms similar to this patient is primary central nervous system lymphoma (PCNSL). PCNSL occurs primarily in the sixth decade of life except for those individuals who are HIV positive when it occurs in the third decade. Patients usually present with cognitive or behavioral changes, headache, or focal symptoms. Seizures are uncommon. PCNSL can be difficult to distinguish on MRI scan from a glial tumor; however, it characteristically involves periventricular structures and usually enhances diffusely and homogeneously. The irregular ring-enhancement of this lobar lesion makes PCNSL less likely. Other primary brain tumors such as a sarcoma or neuronal neoplasm are extremely rare and can only be diagnosed pathologically. They cannot be differentiated from the more common glial tumors on the basis of clinical or radiographic features.

The second category of potential diseases causing an intracranial mass is infection. The triad of symptoms for cerebral abscess is increased intra-cranial pressure, focal deficits, and fever. Seizures or other neurologic symptoms may also occur. There may be an elevated peripheral white blood cell count and erythrocyte sedimentation rate and positive blood cultures if there is a systemic source, but frequently these tests are normal; cerebrospinal fluid (CSF) is usually normal as well. Patients may have a history of head trauma, otitis or sinusitis, cardiac valve disease, or prior neurosurgical or dental procedure any one of which predisposes to brain abscess formation.

The appearance of an abscess on MRI varies according to its age. Late stage or mature abscesses are ring enhancing with a central necrotic region. The ring intensely enhances with contrast but is thinner and more uniform than the enhancement seen in tumors and is often well circumscribed. On T1 abscesses have an isointense center with the capsule being mildly hyperintense. They are hyperintense on T2 with a thin hypointense rim and surrounding edema. They are most commonly seen in the distribution of the middle cerebral artery at the gray–white matter junction, but they can occur anywhere in the brain. Most abscesses are bacterial and they can be polymicrobial in some circumstances. Parasitic, mycobacterial, or fungal infections occur almost exclusively in immunocompromised patients. Their radiographic features are identical to bacterial abscesses although the number, location, and clinical circumstance often suggest the specific diagnosis. Cerebrospinal fluid is nonspecific with elevated protein and mononuclear pleocytosis (<100 cells). In cases of toxoplasmosis, serology is usually positive, unless the patient is too immunocompromised to mount an immune response. Toxoplasmosis lesions occur mostly in the basal ganglia and cervicomedullary junction.

Although a brain abscess is possible, it is an unlikely explanation for this patient's symptoms and signs. He has no predisposing illness or history which makes him vulnerable to a central nervous system infection. He had no constitutional symptoms or evidence of systemic infection at presentation. Furthermore, his right temporoparietal mass is large and has an incomplete enhancing rim which is atypical for an abscess.

The final category of diagnostic possibilities is inflammatory or demyelinating lesions, which can be infectious such as progressive multifocal leukoencephalopathy (PML), postinfectious, or multiple sclerosis (MS). Multifocality is a hallmark of PML, but a single lesion can be seen early in its course. The disease is restricted to white matter where the JC virus, a papova virus, invades oligodendroglia. Radiographically one sees hypointense lesions on T1 MRI images, without surrounding edema on T2 images; the lesions occasionally enhance with contrast. This entity rarely occurs in immunocompetent individuals. Symptoms include lateralizing signs, cognitive dysfunction, visual loss and ataxia. A mild increase in protein concentration and a mild mononuclear pleocytosis may be seen in the CSF. Cerebrospinal fluid polymerase chain reaction for JC virus can be diagnostic. Magnetic resonance imaging findings in Lyme disease can be normal or reveal white matter lesions that are either superficial or deep and may be confluent; some may enhance after contrast administration. Most patients present with symptoms of meningitis, cranial neuritis or radiculoneuritis. Cerebrospinal fluid usually has a lymphocytic pleocytosis with normal to slightly decreased glucose and increased protein concentrations. This patient does not fit the profile of either of these diseases.

Acute disseminated encephalomyelitis is a postinfectious process occurring after vaccination or viral infections, such as an upper respiratory tract infection; neither of these antecedents occurred in this patient. A prodrome of fever, malaise, and myalgias may be the only symptoms prior to the onset of neurologic symptoms and signs. The onset of neurologic disease is rapid and usually manifest by encephalopathy and focal or multifocal symptoms. On MRI multiple subcortical hyperintense white matter lesions are seen on T2 images, some which enhance on T1 after contrast administration. Cerebrospinal fluid is variable but can be normal; oligoclonal bands are usually absent but when present will resolve over time.

Finally, demyelination can present as a single large lesion which mimics a brain tumor. The hallmark of relapsing–remitting MS is multiple lesions distributed in time and space. Patients may have impaired cognition, sensory, motor, or cerebellar function. This patient's past history of optic neuritis makes MS a consideration. Multiple sclerosis primarily affects women in their 20s and 60% of patients with optic neuritis subsequently develop MS. Diagnosis can usually be made by history, imaging studies, evoked potentials, and the presence of oligoclonal bands and elevated immunoglobulin levels in CSF. On MRI, MS plaques are iso-intense to hypointense on T1 and hyperintense on T2. They are usually multiple, periventricular, and they may be confluent. Enhancement is present in acute lesions and may be solid or ring-like. Although this patient has a large partially enhancing mass, no other lesions were evident on his T2 MRI images, making classical MS unlikely.

Diagnostic procedure and treatment

A craniotomy with subtotal resection was performed and the pathologic specimen was interpreted as an anaplastic astrocytoma. The patient then received 6000 cGy of external beam radiotherapy, followed by one cycle of 6-mercaptopurine and lomustine. A repeat MRI scan showed progression of disease and the patient sought alternative opinions. At another institution the pathology was interpreted as demyelination and not tumor. The patient had a lumbar puncture and the CSF was normal. He was treated for presumptive Lyme disease with intravenous ceftriaxone for 4 weeks without any clinical or radiographic improvement. The pathology was reviewed at multiple institutions, all confirming the diagnosis of demyelination.

Further discussion

Treatment for malignant gliomas can increase survival and improve quality of life. The first intervention is surgical resection, if feasible. Patients who have undergone gross total resection survive longer than those who have had a subtotal resection or biopsy only.[1,2] Debulking of the tumor can improve neurologic symptoms and help reduce the requirement for steroids to control edema and symptoms. Post-operatively, all patients with malignant gliomas receive radiotherapy. The standard radiation treatment plan consists of approximately 6000 cGy delivered to the area of the tumor over a course of 6 weeks. Higher doses have been used without increased benefit.[3,4] Adjuvant chemotherapy with nitrosourea can increase the proportion of patients with prolonged survival, but does not improve the median survival.[5,6] The standard prognostic factors of age, performance status, tumor histology and duration of symptoms do not predict benefit from chemotherapy. Because standard chemotherapy is only modestly effective, many patients, including this one, are treated with non-standard regimens or elect to enter experimental protocols.

Extirpation of a brain tumor facilitates diagnosis, decreases mass effect, improves neurologic function, and prolongs survival. When the mass is a demyelinating lesion, resection is usually performed before the correct diagnosis is recognized. Rarely, a neuropathologist may identify demyelination on a frozen section, usually when the clinician suggests this possibility to the pathologist. If demyelination is seen, the surgeon should terminate further removal of tissue. Even when examining permanent sections, the neuropathologist should be alerted to the possibility of demyelination since many of these lesions are misinterpreted as malignant glial tumors. Reactive astrocytes accompany large demyelinating lesions and can be misconstrued as malignant astrocytes, especially in the setting of a large single enhancing lesion on MRI. It is relatively easy to separate the two entities by doing an immunohistochemical assay with the HAM-56 antibody looking for the presence of macrophages, which are not seen in glial tumors. The macrophages within the lesion are filled with myelin breakdown products. A silver stain can delineate the loss of myelin with relative axonal preservation. Other characteristics such as the absence of vascular hyperplasia can be used to recognize demyelination and differentiate it from a malignant glioma.[7] However, reactive lymphocytes and gliosis can be seen in both types of lesions. One characteristic on MRI that may differentiate tumor from a demyelinating lesion is that often the rim of enhancement is thicker and more nodular in high-grade brain tumors than in demyelinating lesions. One report also suggests that demyelinating lesions have an open ring with the incomplete enhancement adjacent to a ventricular surface, as opposed to a closed ring, which is characteristic of neoplasms (Fig. 14.1).[8] Tumors also tend to have more surrounding edema, but this is not helpful in individual cases.

Based on the available literature, it is unclear whether large demyelinating lesions are part of multiple sclerosis or a separate entity. Kepes reviewed 36 cases of large tumor-like demyelinating lesions.[9] In these patients, the age ranged from 10 to 77 years, lesions were primarily solid but some were cystic, and almost all were in the subcortical white matter, not the periventricular region. Symptoms had an acute onset and the lesions disappeared with the use of steroids, without recurrence. Most of the patients had a monophasic illness and never developed a relapsing–remitting or progressive course consistent with MS. These lesions were thought to be more analogous to postinfectious or postvaccination encephalitis than MS. However, it is also clear that some patients with otherwise typical MS develop large lesions, which mimic tumors.

Peterson et al. reviewed five patients who had undergone radiation for suspected primary or metastatic brain tumors,[10] but turned out to have demyelinating lesions instead. Four patients had an idiopathic demyelinating lesion and one had multiple chemotherapy-induced foci of demyelination. All patients had dismal outcomes after treatment with radiotherapy. Radiotherapy has a synergistic effect with demyelination, leading to enhanced destruction of the white matter and a devastating clinical outcome. Radiation can itself lead to demyelination which is occasionally seen as an early delayed toxicity of radiotherapy. Cerebral radiation

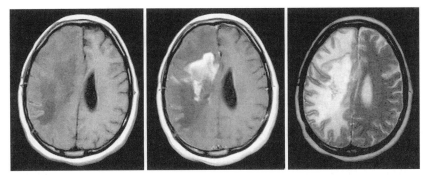

Fig. 14.2. Magnetic resonance imaging carried out 13 months after radiation therapy shows a mass lesion with partial contrast enhancement, mass effect and edema. Left image is T1 without contrast. Middle image is a contrast-enhanced T1. Right image is a T2.

therapy delivered to a patient with a compromised ability to repair central nervous system demyelination injury can lead to severe permanent neurologic dysfunction.

Patient follow-up

At the time of our evaluation, we recommended that the patient pursue physical therapy and taper his dexamethasone. At a dose of 2 mg/day dexamethasone, he began to experience increased headaches, worsening left hemiparesis, and incoordination, necessitating an increase in the corticosteroids. Serial MRI scans showed a progressively enlarging lesion with increased mass effect and contrast enhancement (Fig. 14.2). The patient continued to suffer from raised intracranial pressure and left hemiparesis. He was managed with dexamethasone; 20 months after radiation therapy his symptoms improved and the mass lesion resolved completely on MRI scan (Fig. 14.3). His hemiparesis improved, and his dexamethasone was again tapered.

Diagnosis

Demyelinating mass lesion (probable MS). Radiation-induced white matter injury.

References

1. Ammirati M, Vick N, Liao YL, Ciric I, Mikhael M. Effect of the extent of surgical resection on survival and quality of life in patients with supratentorial glioblastomas and anaplastic astrocytomas. *Neurosurgery* 1987; **21:** 201–206.
2. Winston KR, Walsh JW, Fischer EG. Results of operative treatment of intracranial metastatic tumors. *Cancer* 1980; **45:** 2639–2645.

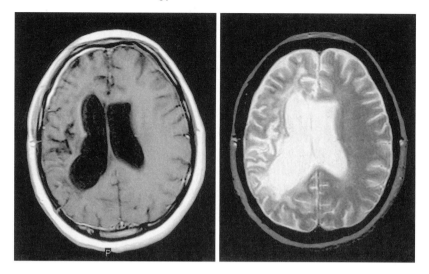

Fig. 14.3. Magnetic resonance imaging carried out 20 months after radiation therapy when symptoms resolved showing cortical atrophy and ex vacuo dilatation of the right lateral ventricle. Left is a contrast-enhanced T1. Right image is a T2.

3. Bleehen NM, Stenning SP. A medical research council trial of two radiotherapy doses in the treatment of grades 3 and 4 astrocytoma. The medical research council brain tumour working party. *Br J Cancer* 1991; **64**: 769–774.

4. Miller PJ, Hassanien RS, Giri PG, Kimler BF, O'Boynick P, Evans RG. Univariate and multivariate statistical analysis of high-grade gliomas: the relationship of radiation dose and other prognostic factors. *Int J Radiat Oncol Biol Phys* 1990; **19**: 275–280.

5. Fine HA, Dear KBG, Loeffler JS, McL Black P., Canellos GP. Meta-analysis of radiation therapy with and without adjuvant chemotherapy for malignant gliomas in adults. *Cancer* 1993; **71**: 2585–2597.

6. DeAngelis LM, Burger PC, Green SB, Cairncross JG. Malignant glioma: who benefits from adjuvant chemotherapy. *Ann Neurol* 1998; **44**, 691–695.

7. Zagzag D, Miller DC, Kleinman GM, Abati A, Donnenfeld H, Budzilovich GN. Demyelinating disease versus tumor in surgical neuropathology. Clues to a correct diagnosis. *Am J Surg Pathol* 1993; **17**: 537–545.

8. Masdeu JC, Moreira J, Trasi S, Visintainer P, Cavaliere R, Grundman M. The open ring. A new imaging sign in demyelinating disease. *J Neuroimaging* 1996; **6**: 104–107.

9. Kepes JJ. Large focal tumor-like demyelinating lesions of the brain: intermediate entity between multiple sclerosis and acute disseminated encephalomyelitis. A study of 31 patients. *Ann Neurol* 1993; **33**: 18–27.

10. Peterson K, Rosenblum MK, Powers JM, Alvord E, Walker RW, Posner JB. Effect of brain irradiation on demyelinating lesions. *Neurology* 1993; **43**: 2105–2112.

A 32-year-old man with progressive spasticity and parkinsonism

Clinical history and examination

A 32-year-old man was referred for evaluation of a 6-year history of spasticity and parkinsonism.

He was adopted at the age of 8 months and birth records were unavailable. He attained normal developmental milestones and graduated from high school. At the age of 22, he worked in a factory where he may have been exposed to solvents (nature, amount and duration of exposure unknown). He quit work after 2 years. He had a history of heavy ethanol use (beginning in high school and ending at the age of 24), occasional marijuana and cocaine use, and a 10-year history of cigarette smoking (one pack per day). There was no history of exposure to neuroleptics and no significant medical history.

At the age of 26, he noted the onset of shaking movements of his left leg. Similar movements subsequently affected his left arm and to a lesser extent his right arm. Movements occurred at rest, were involuntary and rhythmic and could not be suppressed. Changing the position of the extremity would terminate the movements. He and his family next noted insidious onset of slurring of speech. Over the 2 years before evaluation, he became aware of progressive difficulty with coordinated movements. His handwriting deteriorated, becoming sloppy but not overtly micrographic. Fine hand movements became progressively slow and uncoordinated, producing moderate difficulty in cutting food, dressing and performing daily hygiene. At the same time, he became aware of increased difficulty walking. Family and friends noted that he was slower and less stable, tending to walk with a mild shuffle with stooped posture and leaning to one side. He was aware of a change in arm position when walking, usually keeping his arms immobile in a flexed posture.

The patient did not have urinary, bowel or erectile dysfunction and had no lightheadedness on standing. He had multiple dental infections, requiring the removal of virtually all of his upper teeth. Despite a good appetite, his oral intake was decreased, and he sustained an 80 lb weight loss over the 4 years prior to evaluation. The patient and his sister did not think that his cognitive status had changed significantly. In particular, he did not have memory loss, hallucinations or abnormal behaviors. He lived alone and required assistance only for transportation and shopping.

General physical examination was unremarkable. Seated blood pressure was 140/90 mmHg without change on standing.

Neurologic examination revealed significant deficits in mental status. He was alert and oriented, followed complex commands and had preserved language ability (reading, writing, naming, repetition). However, he was unable to perform serial 7s or serial 3s and could not perform simple calculations. Short-term and long-term memory was moderately impaired. He was able to name the months of the year forward but only partially in reverse. Although aware of these difficulties, he was unconcerned by them. His speech was mildly hypophonic and moderately dysarthric. His vocabulary was limited (relative to expected baseline). He was passive during examination, waiting for the examiner to ask questions and then answering in short phrases.

Cranial nerve examination revealed bilaterally equal, round and reactive pupils. His fundoscopic examination was normal, as were confrontational visual fields. No Kayser–Fleischer rings were present. Extraocular movements were quick and full on saccade and pursuit. There were no square wave jerks, and opticokinetic nystagmus was normal in both the horizontal and vertical directions. Moderate facial masking and depressed blink rate was seen. Volitional and emotional facial movements were slow, as were his tongue movements. The remainder of the cranial nerve examination was unremarkable.

Motor and coordination examination revealed full power and no atrophy or fasciculations. Mild spasticity and marked cogwheeling were present at the neck and in the limbs, worse on the left than the right. There was marked slowing and decrement in amplitude of fine hand and foot movements. Intermittent rhythmic clonic movements of 3–4 Hz frequently affected the left leg and arms. Movements were suppressed by changing the position of the arm and leg. There were no myoclonic or choreic movements.

Sensory examination revealed intact primary sensory modalities bilaterally. He was able to arise from a seated position without arm assistance. His gait was slightly unsteady with decreased arm swing. Stride was quick, but turning was slightly slow. He kept his left arm flexed and held close to his torso. Recovery on pull test was normal. Reflexes were extremely brisk with several beats of clonus triggered in both upper and lower extremities.

Finger flexor jerks, snout reflex, Hoffmans and Myersons signs were prominent with bilateral Babinskis. Jaw jerk was extremely brisk, occasionally eliciting sustained clonus.

A brief trial of Sinemet (maximum dose 25/250 mg three times daily) produced no improvement in his symptoms or examination. It was discontinued because of nausea.

Routine serum chemistries and a complete blood count were within normal limits. Creatine kinase was normal and careful examination of his peripheral smear did not show acanthocytes. Slit lamp examination revealed no Kayser–Fleischer rings and his retinae were normal. Serum ceruloplasmin was 31 mg/dl (normal 25–63 mg/dl). An electromyogram and skin and muscle biopsy was performed and were normal. No ragged red fibers were seen and there was no evidence of a neurogenic or myopathic process. A lysosomal batter (including beta-galactosidase and hexosaminidase A) was normal.

An MRI of the head was performed (Fig. 15.1), showing mild cerebral atrophy, moderate atrophy of the striatum, and increased signal within the putamen on long spin echo images (T2 and proton density). No calcifications or accumulations of iron were seen. A diagnostic test was performed.

$$* \qquad * \qquad *$$

Discussion

This 32-year-old man presented with a 6-year course of insidious and unrelenting spasticity and parkinsonism. Aside from a history of exposure to unknown solvents, severe dental caries and an 80 lb weight loss, few additional historical clues were available to suggest the diagnosis. As an adopted child, his family history was unknown.

Neurologic examination revealed a subcortical dementia with apathy, inattention and inability to concentrate out of proportion to preserved cortical abilities. There were no gross abnormalities of the oculomotor system. Prominent axial and appendicular spasticity and parkinsonism dominated the examination. Spasticity was impressive, with sustained clonus of the leg mimicking tremor, and clonus of the jaw which could be entrained on occasion for periods as long as 30 seconds.

Laboratory studies, including creatine kinase, peripheral blood smear for acanthocytes, slit lamp examination for Kayser–Fleischer rings, serum ceruloplasmin, lysosomal battery, EMG, and skin and muscle biopsy were normal. The only study which was abnormal, and which ultimately led to the diagnosis, was the MRI of the head – it will be discussed.

The differential diagnosis of a young individual with parkinsonism, spasticity and cognitive decline is broad. Among the major categories to consider are toxin exposure, infectious and para-infectious disorders,

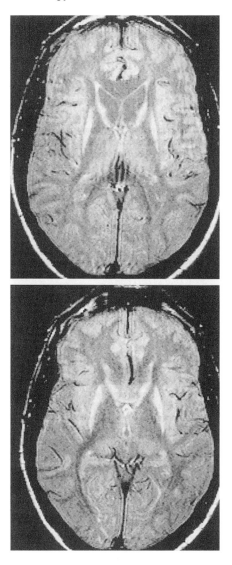

Fig. 15.1. Adjacent axial proton-dense images are shown. Mild cerebral atrophy and moderate striatal atrophy are present. Increased signal is present bilaterally in the putamen.

metabolic disorders and neurodegenerative illnesses. These will be considered in turn below.

This patient's history is notable for a 2-year exposure to unknown solvents. A large number of toxins can cause parkinsonism, including manganese, mercury, hydrocarbons and MPTP.[1-3] However, none of these agents cause the characteristic signal changes seen on this patient's MRI. Although systemic infection with HIV can cause a variety of movement disorders, the time course of the illness is inconsistent with this disorder. Similar comments apply to paraneoplastic parkinsonism, an infrequent cause of parkinsonism.[4]

Among the metabolic disorders, Wilsons disease should be considered in the differential diagnosis of any young person presenting with a movement disorder. This patient's clinical profile is consistent with Wilsons disease, as the protean manifestations of this disorder include dysarthria, tremor, dystonia, spasticity and cognitive change.[5] Increased signal on long Tr images is also common in this condition, although selective involvement of the putamen would be highly unusual.[6] Although a 24-hour urinary copper collection was not performed, the absence of Kayser–Fleischer rings on slit lamp exam and a normal ceruloplasmin make this diagnosis extremely unlikely.

Leighs disease should be considered in the differential diagnosis, particularly given the appearance of the MRI. This disorder typically affects children, although adult-onset cases have been reported. Adult patients typically present with global cognitive and motor decline and an elevated serum or cerebrospinal fluid lactate.[7] The absence of ragged red fibers on muscle biopsy does not automatically exclude this diagnosis.

Other rarer possibilities include neuroacanthocytosis and Hallervorden–Spatz disease. A normal creatine kinase and peripheral smear argue against the first possibility. Hallervorden–Spatz disease can present with dystonia and parkinsonism in adulthood, although the characteristic iron deposition within the basal ganglia is not seen in this patient's MRI.[8] Lysosomal studies were also normal, ruling out an unusual adult presentation of a childhood storage disorder.

Ultimately, the appearance of the MRI led to the correct diagnosis. The presence of high signal in the putamen, accompanied by caudate and putaminal atrophy suggested the possibility of Huntingtons disease. This was also supported by the history of early adoption (sometimes indicative of parental distress or instability) and a profound unexplained weight loss. A direct gene test for CAG expansions within the IT-15 (Huntingtons disease) gene was performed. This test revealed the diagnosis: one normal allele (19 repeats) and one abnormal expanded allele (47 repeats).

Huntingtons disease, an autosomal dominant disorder with 100% penetrance, is caused by expansion of CAG repeats in the IT-15 gene above a critical level (37–40 repeats). Patients with larger repeat size develop symptoms earlier and deteriorate more rapidly. When paternally inherited, there is a greater risk of expansion of repeat size. Although typically beginning between the ages of 35 and 45, early symptoms of Huntingtons disease (chorea, cognitive decline and personality change) can begin as early as the first and as late as the ninth decade.[9] Dysarthria, dysphagia, gait disturbance and weight loss are also common.[10] Although many Huntingtons disease patients have eye movement abnormalities, eye movements can be normal even in advanced cases.[11] In 2 years of follow-up since the diagnosis, the patient has developed slowing of voluntary saccades and a tendency to blink when generating a saccade, an abnormality seen in 35% of Huntington patients.[11]

Our patient's MRI contained two clues to the diagnosis: striatal atrophy and symmetric increased signal in the putamen on long Tr images. Atrophy of the caudate and increased bicaudate ratio are well-known features of Huntingtons disease[12] and were often used for diagnosis before the availability of genetic testing. However, atrophy of the putamen is a more sensitive marker for early Huntingtons disease.[13] Increase in signal on long Tr images may be seen in Wilsons disease,[6] Leighs disease[7] and other disorders. However, it would be very unusual for the putamen to be selectively involved in these conditions. On the other hand, increased putaminal signal has been reported in Huntingtons disease,[14-17] and is associated with early-onset and increased severity of disability.[14]

Early descriptions of Huntingtons disease classified patients by clinical phenotype. A rigid adult variant, dominated by spasticity, parkinsonism, dystonia and cognitive decline was first described by Westphal and later by Hamilton.[18] Juvenile Huntingtons disease (with onset of symptoms before the age of 20) typically resembles the rigid variant with additional features of seizures and cerebellar findings.[18] However, these classifications are artificial. Large clinical series have confirmed that neurologic features of Huntingtons disease are best viewed as a continuum. Among 624 patients with the disease, Farrer and Conneally demonstrated a continuous progression of symptoms with an inverse relationship between rigidity and rate of disease progression to age of symptom onset.[18] A review of 195 cases of juvenile Huntingtons disease from the world literature[19] and 53 cases from the Netherlands[20] confirmed that juvenile Huntington patients are not clinically distinct from other patients, but instead represent a severe and early form of the illness.

Treatment of the akinetic–rigid form of Huntingtons disease is limited. Patients may respond to levodopa[21] but often they do not. Exacerbation of chorea or the development of psychosis[22] may limit the utility of this treatment. Subsequent trials of tizanidine, baclofen, and gabapentin were similarly unhelpful in this patient. Unfortunately, effective pharmacologic agents for akinetic–rigid Huntingtons disease are currently unavailable.

Diagnosis

Huntingtons disease.

This chapter was originally published with a videotape of the patient as a Clinical Grand Rounds in Movement Disorders (1999; Volume 14, pages 350–357). The text has been slightly altered to fit the format of this book.

References

1. Huang CC, Chu NS, Lu CS, Chen RS, Calne DB. Long-term progression in chronic manganism: 10 years of follow-up. *Neurology* 1998; **50:** 698–700.
2. Finkelstein Y, Vardi J, Kesten MM, Hod I. The enigma of parkinsonism in chronic borderline mercury intoxication, resolved by challenge with penicillamine. *Neurotoxicology* 1996; **17:** 291–295.
3. Langston JW, Ballard P, Tetrud JW, Irwin I. Chronic parkinsonism in humans due to a product of meperidine analogue synthesis. *Science* 1983; **219:** 979–980.
4. Golbe LI, Miller DC, Duvoisin RC. Paraneoplastic degeneration of the substantia nigra with dystonia and parkinsonism. *Mov Disord* 1989; **4:** 147–152.
5. Walshe JM, Yealland M. Wilsons disease: the problem of delayed diagnosis. *J Neurol Neurosurg Psychiatry* 1992; **55:** 692–696.
6. Saatci I, Topcu M, Baltaoglu FF et al. Cranial MR findings in Wilsons disease. *Acta Radiologica* 1997; **38:** 250–258.
7. Rahman S, Blok RB, Kahl H-HM et al. Leigh syndrome: clinical features and biochemical and DNA abnormalities. *Ann Neurol* 1996; **39:** 343–351.
8. Swaiman KF. Hallervorden-Spatz syndrome and brain iron metabolism. *Arch Neurol* 1991; **48:** 1285–1293.
9. Marshall FJ, Shoulson I. Clinical features and treatment of Huntingtons disease. In: Watts RL, Koller WC, eds. *Movement Disorders*. New York: McGraw-Hill, 1997: 491–502.
10. Farrer LA, Conneally PM. Predictability of phenotype in Huntingtons disease. *Arch Neurol* 1987; **44:** 109–113.
11. Lasker AG, Zee DS. Ocular motor abnormalities in Huntingtons disease. *Vision Res* 1997; **37:** 3639–3645.
12. Aylward EH, Li Q, Stine OC et al. Longitudinal change in basal ganglia volume in patients with Huntingtons disease. *Neurology* 1997; **48:** 394–399.
13. Harris GJH, Pearlson GD, Peyser CE et al. Putamen volume reduction on magnetic resonance imaging exceeds caudate changes in mild Huntingtons disease. *Ann Neurol* 1992; **31:** 69–75.
14. Oliva D, Carella F, Savoiardo M et al. Clinical and magnetic resonance features of the classic and akinetic–rigid variants of Huntingtons disease. *Arch Neurol* 1993; **50:** 17–19.
15. Sethi KD. Magnetic resonance imaging in Huntingtons disease. *Mov Disord* 1991; **6:** 186.
16. Spieker S, Petersen D, Poremba M. MRI in a case of rigid Huntingtons disease. *J Neurol Neurosurg Psychiatry* 1993; **56:** 834–845.
17. Kang UJ, Fahn S, Schwarz H, Shoulson I, Vallejos H, Goldman J. What is it? Case 1: 1989: juvenile-onset parkinsonism, dystonia, and pyramidal tract signs. *Mov Disord* 1989; **4:** 363–370.
18. Farrer LA, Conneally PM. Predictability of phenotype in Huntingtons disease. *Arch Neurol* 1987; **44:** 109–113.
19. van Dijk JG, van der Velde EA, Roos RAC, Bruyn GW. Juvenile Huntingtons disease. *Hum Genet* 1986; **73:** 235–239.
20. Siesling S, Veget-van der Vlis M, Roos RAC. Juvenile Huntingtons disease in the Netherlands. *Pediatr Neurol* 1997; **17:** 37–43.
21. Barbeau A. L-dopa and juvenile Huntingtons disease. *Lancet* 1969; **2:** 1066.
22. Low PA, Allsop JL, Halmagyi GM. Huntingtons chorea: the rigid form (Westphal variant) treated with levodopa. *Med J Aust* 1974; **1:** 393–394.

Acute confusion

Clinical history and examination

A 66-year-old man was admitted to the hospital because of altered mentation.

Except for a past history of peptic ulcer, he was well until 2 days prior to admission, when he acutely developed headache, nausea, and vomiting and then felt as if he were 'losing his mind.' His memory was impaired and he experienced strange visual symptoms, variably describing diplopia or polyopia, inability to recognize faces, and metamorphopsia; objects, for example, automobiles, appeared decreased in length and increased in height. There were neither weakness nor sensory symptoms.

He was right-handed, spoke only Spanish, worked as a cook, and lived alone. He smoked a pack of cigarettes and drank two beers daily for over 20 years; he denied other recreational drug use. He took cimetidine for peptic ulcer symptoms. His mother and father were deceased but he could not say at what age or what caused death. He had completed seventh grade. He required glasses for reading. Review of systems was otherwise negative, including psychiatric symptoms.

The temperature was 98°F, pulse 80 per minute and regular, respirations 16 per minute and regular, and blood pressure 120/80 mmHg. There was no evidence of head trauma. A grade 2/6 systolic murmur was heard over the left upper sternal border without radiation. No carotid bruits were present, and examination of the heart and lungs was otherwise normal, as was the rest of the general physical examination.

On neurological examination he was alert and cooperative but complaining of difficulty thinking clearly, and the details of his recent history were at times contradictory and implausible. (For example, in one version he described his symptoms occurring shortly after a friend gave him 'some medicine' to drink.) He was intermittently inattentive and abulic, with a paucity of spontaneous speech and an inappropriate lack of concern for his condition. He was able to count backward from 20 to 1, but his performance was hesitant. He was oriented to person and year but not to month or day of the week, and he repeatedly gave the wrong name of the hospital he was in. He knew that Clinton was the President and that President Kennedy's son had recently died in a plane crash, yet he had difficulty recalling how many children he had. He correctly named objects and wrote a dictated sentence. He did not have his glasses and would not attempt to read or to copy diagrams without them. He could perform simple calculations, and there was no hemineglect or apraxia. Except for an (uncorrected) visual acuity of 20/200 bilaterally, the rest of the neurological examination was normal, including fundi, gross visual fields, other cranial nerves, strength, coordination, gait, sensation, and reflexes.

The hematocrit was 45% and the white blood cell count was $10\,800/mm^3$, with 74% neutrophils, 13% lymphocytes, 12% monocytes, and 1% eosinophils. The platelet count was $215\,000/mm^3$. The erythrocyte sedimentation rate was 43 mm/h. The urine contained 'few' white blood cells and 'trace' protein; the urine was positive for cocaine metabolites and negative for amphetamines, barbiturates, methadone, opiates, benzodiazepines, cannabinoids, and phencyclidine. Blood glucose, blood urea nitrogen, and serum creatinine, sodium, potassium, chloride, bicarbonate, calcium, conjugated and total bilirubin, total protein, albumin, alkaline phosphatase, aspartate aminotransferase, and uric acid were normal. Prothrombin time was 11.9 seconds (INR 1.06). Partial thromboplastin time was 28.15 seconds. Serum cholesterol was 243 mg/dl. Cerebrospinal fluid had normal appearance and pressure and contained one white blood cell and 55 red blood cells/mm^3; CSF protein was 19 mg/dl and glucose was 76 mg/dl. The CSF was negative for cryptococcal antigen. Serum and CSF syphilis screen (RPR) were nonreactive. Serum thyroid-stimulating hormone, thyroxine, and cobalamin were normal. Antinuclear antibodies were not present.

An electrocardiogram was normal. Computed tomographic (CT) scan of the head revealed bilateral occipitoparietal and left frontal hypodensities suggestive of infarction. Magnetic resonance imaging revealed bilateral occipitoparietal wedge-shaped areas of increased signal on long-TR sequences consistent with either border-zone infarcts or embolic events (Fig. 16.1). A left frontal subcortical infarct was also present, and there were multiple bilateral focal areas of high signal in the periventricular and subcortical white matter suggestive of ischemic changes. The cerebral ventricles and sulci were prominent, consistent with mild atrophy. Magnetic resonance angiography revealed normal cervical and intracranial vessels.

He was treated with clopidogrel, and the next day his examination was unchanged. Attempts to reach family members, friends, or his employer were unsuccessful. A diagnostic procedure was performed.

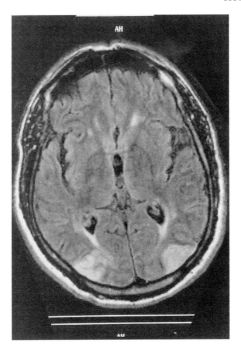

Fig. 16.1. Magnetic resonance imaging showing bilateral occipitoparietal lesions, plus left subcortical and multiple periventricular lesions, consistent with infarction. (Courtesy Dr Paoula Bowers.)

*   *   *

Discussion

Over 2 days this 66-year-old man became severely encephalopathic, with inattentiveness, psychomotor slowing, impaired memory, and, by his own description, peculiar visual distortions and possibly prosopagnosia, the inability to recognize faces. Typical of an amnestic disturbance, he could immediately register information, and his memory for recent information was more impaired than for remote information, but the dissociation was inconsistent, as reflected in his recall of certain current news events while expressing uncertainty about his own more remote past. Abrupt memory impairment of this sort can be a consequence of structural lesions, usually bilateral, involving the limbic system, especially the inferomedial temporal lobe or the medial thalamus; such might be seen with herpes simplex encephalitis or cerebrovascular disease affecting the posterior circulation. Abrupt memory impairment can also be the consequence of head trauma, intoxication, seizure, or any of a large number of metabolic derangements. When the features of amnesia are bizarre – for example, loss of personal identity with preservation of recent memory – a psychiatric origin is more likely.

The patient's visual symptoms suggest a disturbance of visual associative areas. Metamorphopsia (occasionally encountered as a seizure aura) and prosopagnosia suggest occipitotemporal pathology; with prosopagnosia bilateral lesions were likely. Whether his poor visual acuity simply reflected refractive error or was partly the result of lesions affecting central visual pathways is uncertain, for corrected visual acuity was not determined.

Altered mentation unaccompanied by motor, sensory, or other abnormalities on examination raise the suspicion of CNS infection, metabolic derangement, or intoxication, and, indeed, cocaine metabolites were present in the urine. Cocaine intoxication, however, lasts minutes to hours, not days, and produces psychosis or delirium, not a predominantly amnestic disorder, and there is often hyperthermia, hypertension, and metabolic acidosis. Moreover, CT and later MRI showed structural lesions attributed to multiple infarcts in both cerebral hemispheres.

Multiple ischemic strokes can be a consequence of CNS infection, especially tuberculous meningitis; such patients usually have obvious systemic illness and delirium or stupor, and a spinal tap performed on this man revealed normal CSF.

Ischemic strokes, sometimes multiple, are also associated with cocaine use, especially smokable alkaloidal 'crack.' Although one case-control study did not identify cocaine use as a risk factor for stroke,[1] a large number of anecdotal reports and case series involving young people without other risk factors argue in favor of causality. To date, more than 400 cases of cocaine-related stroke have been reported, roughly half hemorrhagic and half ischemic.[2] Hemorrhagic strokes, often occurring in the presence of underlying saccular aneurysms or vascular malformations, are probably the result of acute hypertension. Ischemic strokes might be secondary to cocaine-induced cerebral vasospasm and abetted by effects of the drug on platelets and coagulation factors. Cardioembolic stroke has been blamed on cocaine-induced cardiomyopathy and could theoretically be a complication of cocaine-induced myocardial infarction. The extent of this patient's cocaine use was uncertain – he denied using the drug at all – and although the appearance of his infarcts on CT and MRI suggested embolism, there was no evidence of cardiac disease.

A number of uncommon diseases need to be considered in the presence of multiple brain infarcts. Granulomatous angiitis of the nervous system affects small ($<200\,\mu$m diameter) leptomeningeal arteries and veins, with segmental mononuclear and granulomatous lesions.[3] It occurs in patients with herpes zoster, lymphoma, or sarcoidosis but most often is not associated with any underlying disorder. Headache and altered mentation usually precede focal signs such as hemiparesis. The CSF may be normal or have lymphocytic pleocytosis and elevated protein content.

Cerebral angiography may be normal or show segmental vessel narrowing ('beading'), which, however, is not specific for vasculitis. Untreated, the disease is usually fatal, with survival lasting days to years. Anecdotal reports favor treatment with corticosteroids and immunosuppressants.

Lymphomatoid granulomatosis, in which vessels are infiltrated with lymphoreticular cells and display necrosis and granuloma formation, typically affects the lungs, with CNS involvement in approximately one-third of cases. Restriction of the disease to the nervous system is rare, and symptoms, which do not usually present as frank stroke, may be misdiagnosed as encephalitis or multiple sclerosis.[4]

In neoplastic angioendotheliomatosis atypical mononuclear cells are present in small blood vessels of many organs. Skin and CNS involvement are most likely to be symptomatic, and progressive dementia, impaired memory, or aphasia may be prominent. Malignant intravascular lymphoma has been proposed as an alternative name for this disease, which is usually fatal within a few months to a few years.[5]

Venous sinus or cortical venous thrombosis can produce bilateral infarcts, often hemorrhagic. An underlying process such as a parameningeal infection or a hematologic disorder (or, in women, pregnancy or the use of oral contraceptives) is often present.[6]

Although usually associated with lobar intracerebral hemorrhage, amyloid angiopathy can cause multiple cortical infarcts. The patient's age qualifies him for that diagnosis. Amyloid angiopathy tends to affect small arteries, however, producing microinfarcts found incidentally at autopsies of subjects dying of intracerebral hemorrhage.[7]

As noted, the MRI and CT appearance of the lesions was considered most consistent with either border zone ('watershed') or embolic infarction. Bilateral border zone infarction suggests a period of severe hypotension, which was not a feature of the patient's history. Bilateral embolic infarction, affecting both the occipital and frontal lobes, suggests a cardiac or systemic source rather than embolism from disease of the carotid, vertebral, or basilar arteries. Atrial fibrillation was not present, there were no signs on examination of valvular disease or congestive heart failure, and there were no symptoms or electrocardiographic evidence of myocardial infarction. Other possible embolic sources include atrial myxoma (which would likely be associated with systemic symptoms), non-bacterial thrombotic endocarditis (usually associated with cancer, especially adenocarcinoma, but also reported as a complication of AIDS), systemic thrombophlebitis in the presence of a patent foramen ovale, and atherosclerosis of the aortic arch. Favoring the latter would be the patient's elevated serum cholesterol level and the absence of apparent cardiac disease.

An appropriate diagnostic study at this point would have been ultrasound examination of the heart and aortic arch.

The chemical diagnosis was multiple cerebral infarcts, probably secondary to embolism from a cardiac or systemic source.

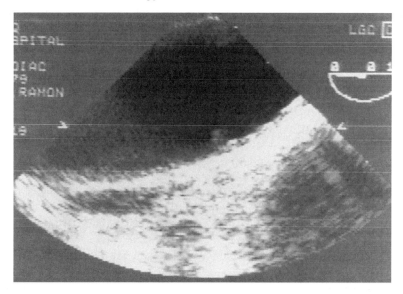

Fig. 16.2. Transesophageal echocardiography showing a mobile atheromatous plaque in the transverse arch of the aorta. (Courtesy Dr Erik Vanderbush.)

Findings and discussion

Transesophageal echocardiography (TEE) revealed a mobile atheromatous plaque in the transverse arch of the aorta (Fig. 16.2). There was diffusely hypokinetic left ventricular function during systole and calcification of the aortic valve with mild aortic stenosis. No right-to-left shunt was seen with agitated saline contrast.

Case-control studies reveal that atherosclerotic plaques in the aortic arch are independent risk factors for brain ischemia.[8-14] For example, in an autopsy study of 500 consecutive patients at the Salpêtrière Hospital in Paris, ulcerated plaques in the aortic arch were found in 28% of patients with cerebrovascular disease and only 5% of those with other neurological disease, for an odds ratio of 4.0.[9] Among those with 'brain infarct of unknown cause' the odds ratio was 5.7, and the presence of ulcerated plaques in the aortic arch did not correlate with the presence of carotid artery stenosis or atrial fibrillation. Ninety-seven per cent of patients with ulcerated plaques in the aortic arch were 60 years of age or older. In a study of TEE in patients with ischemic stroke of unknown cause, the presence of plaques with a mobile component was associated with a risk ratio of 14.[8]

In a prospective study of 331 consecutive patients followed for 2–4 years after brain infarction, the incidence of recurrent brain infarction per 100 person-years was 2.8 in patients with no aortic plaques, 3.5 in those with plaques less than 4 mm in thickness, 11.9 in those with plaques 4 mm or greater in thickness, and 16.4 in those with brain infarction of unknown cause and plaques 4 mm or greater in thickness.[15] The same study showed that aortic plaques also predicted coronary artery and peripheral vascular disease. Embolism from aortic plaques probably accounts for some cerebrovascular events associated with cerebral angiography, aortography, cardiac catheterization, and coronary angioplasty.[16,17] Whereas the major risk factor for carotid stenosis is hypertension, the major risk factor for aortic atherosclerosis is cigarette smoking.[12,14,15]

Emboli from aortic plaques can be composed of cholesterol crystals or thrombotic material. Cholesterol emboli tend to occlude small (< 200 μm) distal arteries and can produce fluctuating or progressive neurological symptoms, sometimes predominantly mental.[18] Recurrent cholesterol emboli have produced a border zone distribution of infarction.[19,20] Systemic organ involvement often coexists. It has been suggested that anticoagulation or thrombolytic therapy might increase the risk of cholesterol embolism from aortic plaques by preventing thrombus formation over plaque ulceration.[21,22]

In contrast to cholesterol emboli, thromboemboli from aortic plaques are more likely to occlude larger cerebral vessels. Suspected risk factors for thrombus formation include plaque rupture, hypercoagulable state, and anticardiolipin antibodies.[23,24]

Uncontrolled studies suggest that anticoagulation and antiplatelet therapy are both of benefit in patients with aortic plaques.[15,25] Although definitive data are lacking, at least a short course of anticoagulation therapy is preferred for mobile thrombi in the lumen of the aortic arch.[26] Other treatment approaches include aortic resection and grafting,[27] endarterectomy,[24,28] and thrombolysis.[29]

Clinical follow-up

The patient received heparin and warfarin. Over the next few days his conversation and motor activity became more animated, and he no longer experienced diplopia or visual distortions. His memory remained poor, however. Diffusion-weighted MRI revealed that the right occipito-parietal lesion was acute and that the other lesions were not (Fig. 16.3). Doppler ultrasonography revealed normal cervical vessels.

Diagnosis

Embolic cerebral infarction secondary to atherosclerosis of the aortic arch.

References

1. Qureshi AL, Akber MS, Czander E et al. Crack cocaine use and stroke in young patients. *Neurology* 1997; **48:** 341–345.
2. Brust JCM. Stroke and substance abuse. In Barnett HJM, Mohr JP, Stein BM, Yatsu FM, eds. *Stroke: Pathophysiology, Diagnosis, and Management.* New York: Churchill-Livingstone, 1998: 979–1000.

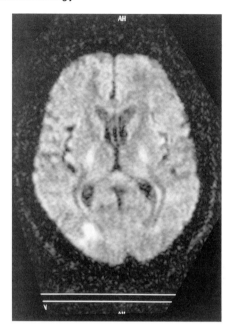

Fig. 16.3. Diffusion-weighted MRI showing an acute right-sided occipitoparietal infarct. (Courtesy Dr Paoula Bowers.)

3. Younger DS, Hayes A., Brust JCM, Rowland LP. Granulamatous angiitis of the brain. An inflammatory reaction of diverse etiology. *Arch Neurol* 1988; **45:** 514–518.
4. Schmidt BJ, Meagher-Villemure K, Del Carpio J. Lymphomatoid granulomatosis with isolated involvement of the brain. *Ann Neurol* 1984; **15:** 478–481.
5. Carroll TJJ, Schelper RL, Goeken JA et al. Naming 'malignant angioendotheliomatosis'. *N Engl J Med* 1986; **315:** 895–896.
6. Ameri A, Bousser MG. Cerebral venous thrombosis. *Neurol Clin* 1992; **10:** 87–111.
7. Greenberg SM, Vonsattel JPG, Stakes JW et al. The clinical spectrum of cerebral amyloid angiopathy: presentation without lobar hemorrhage. *Neurology* 1993; **43:** 2073–2079.
8. Amarenco P, Cohen A, Tzourio C et al. Atherosclerotic disease of the aortic arch and the risk of ischemic stroke. *N Engl J Med* 1994; **331:** 1474–1479.
9. Amarenco P, Duyckaerts C, Tzourio C et al. The prevalence of ulcerated plaques in the aortic arch in patients with stroke. *N Engl J Med* 1992; **326:** 221–225.
10. Khathibzadeh M, Mitusch R, Stierle U et al. Aortic atherosclerotic plaques as a source of systemic embolism. *J Am Coll Cardiol* 1996; **27:** 664–669.
11. Tunick PA, Perez JL, Kronzon I. Protruding atheromas in the thoracic aorta and systemic embolization. *Ann Intern Med* 1991; **115:** 423–427.
12. Jones EF, Kalman JM, Calafiore P et al. Proximal aortic atheroma. An independent risk factor for cerebral ischemia. *Stroke* 1995; **26:** 218–224.

13. DiTullio MR, Sacco RL, Gersony D et al. Aortic atheromas and acute ischemic stroke: a transesophageal echocardiographic study in an ethnically mixed population. *Neurology* 1996; **46:** 1560–1566.

14. Dávila-Román VG, Barzilai B, Wareing TH et al. Atherosclerosis of the ascending aorta. Prevalence and role as independent predictor of cerebrovascular events in cardiac patients. *Stroke* 1994; **25:** 2010–2016.

15. The French Study of Aortic Plaques in Stroke Group: atherosclerotic disease of the aortic arch as a risk factor for recurrent ischemic stroke. *N Engl J Med* 1996; **334:** 1216–1221.

16. Ramirez G, O'Neill WM, Lambert R, Bloomer A. Cholesterol embolization, a complication of angiography. *Arch Intern Med* 1978; **138:** 1430–1432.

17. Wang SP, Chiang BN. Thrombus formation in the ascending aorta: a complication of angiography. *Cathet Cardiovasc Diagn* 1987; **13:** 50–53.

18. McDonald WI. Recurrent cholesterol embolism as a cause of fluctuating cerebral symptoms. *J Neurol Neurosurg Psychiatry* 1967; **30:** 489–496.

19. Case records of the Massachusetts General Hospital. *N Engl J Med* 1967; 276: 1368–1377.

20. Beal MF, Williams RS, Richardson EP, Fisher CM. Cholesterol embolism as a cause of transient ischemic attacks and cerebral infarction. *Neurology* 1981; **31:** 860–865.

21. Oster P, Rieben FW, Waldherr R, Schettler G. Blood clotting and cholesterol crystal embolization. *JAMA* 1979; **242:** 2070–2071.

22. Mendia R, Cavaliere G, Sparacio F et al. Does thrombolysis produce cholesterol embolization? *Lancet* 1992; **339:** 562.

23. Shapiro ME, Rodvien R, Bauer KA, Salzman EW. Acute aortic thrombosis in antithrombine-III deficiency. *JAMA* 1988; **245:** 1759–1761.

24. Tunick PA, Lackner H, Katz ES et al. Multiple emboli from a large aortic arch thrombus in a patient with thrombotic diathesis. *Am Heart J* 1992; **124:** 239–241.

25. Mitusch R, Doherty C, Wucherpfennig H et al. Vascular events during follow-up in patients with aortic arch atherosclerosis. *Stroke* 1997; **28:** 36–39.

26. Amarenco P, Cohen A. Atherosclerotic disease of the aortic arch. In Barnett HJM, Mohr JP, Yatsu F, Stein B, eds. *Stroke: Pathophysiology, Diagnosis, and Treatment*, 3rd edn. Philadelphia: Churchill-Livingstone, 1998: 895–919.

27. Belden JF, Caplan LR, Bojar R et al. Treatment of multiple brain emboli from an ulcerated, thrombogenic aorta with aortectomy and graft replacement. *Neurology* 1997; **49:** 621–622.

28. Tunick PA, Culliford AT, Lamparello PJ, Kronzon I. Atheromatosis of the aortic arch as an occult source of multiple systemic emboli. *Ann Intern Med* 1991; **114:** 391–392.

29. Hausmann D, Golba D, Bargheer K et al. Successful thrombolysis of an aortic arch thrombus in a patient after mesenteric embolism. *N Engl J Med* 1992; **327:** 500–501.

Rapidly progressive weakness

Clinical history and examination

A 32-year-old, right-handed man was admitted to the hospital because of rapidly progressive muscle weakness.

Two days before admission he developed severe back pain in the interscapular region and also pain in his legs. The pain worsened through the night. Early the next morning, he became aware of a tingling sensation in his feet which rapidly spread to involve his hands and then his face in a circumoral distribution. The same day he noticed weakness in his legs, particularly climbing stairs. By the day of admission, he was unable to walk unaided and had difficulty maintaining a sitting position. There was no disturbance of sphincter function.

Two weeks previously he had experienced a bout of acute gastroenteritis, characterized mainly by diarrhea with some abdominal pain, which took several days to settle. There was no other past medical history of note.

He had no family history of neuromuscular disease. A non-smoker, he drank alcohol in moderation. There was no history of exposure to trauma or toxic materials. He had arrived in the UK from Canada on a business trip 4 weeks previously. There was no other significant recent history of travel. He was not taking any regular medication and had no known allergies.

The temperature was 37°C, the pulse was 80 per minute and the respirations were 16 per minute. The blood pressure was 160/90 mmHg.

Neurological examination on admission revealed normal cognitive function and speech. Fundoscopy was normal with no evidence of papilledema. The remainder of the cranial nerve examination was also normal. Examination of the limbs showed normal muscle bulk and tone. There was symmetrical weakness of the upper and lower limbs, MRC grade 3/5 throughout. Coordination was normal within the constraints imposed by his muscle weakness. He was tendon areflexic, plantar responses were flexor. Sensory testing revealed impaired vibration sense in the feet but no other deficits despite his symptoms. He was unable to walk unaided.

Examination of the cardiovascular and respiratory systems, and the abdomen, was normal. His vital capacity on admission was 5.6 liters.

He continued to deteriorate in hospital. The day after admission, his arms became weaker and his swallowing was judged unsafe. His vital capacity fell to 4.6 liters. The next day it was 3.5 liters and he had hypertensive episodes, to a systolic pressure of 170 mmHg. His limbs were weaker and he had a weak cough and gag reflex. He was transferred from the neurology ward to the intensive therapy unit for closer observation. Later the same day, the vital capacity fell progressively to 2.2 liters. He was electively intubated and assisted ventilation was commenced for his worsening bulbar and respiratory muscle weakness. By this time, muscle power in his limbs was 0-1/5.

Routine hematological and biochemical investigations, including full blood count, erythrocyte sedimentation rate, serum urea, electrolytes, calcium, magnesium, glucose and liver function were normal on admission. Over the next few days, minor abnormalities of liver function developed, specifically modest elevation of transaminases, and his serum sodium fell below 130 mmol/l. Creatine kinase was mildly elevated.

Arterial blood gases were normal on admission. Thyroid function, syphilis, *Borrelia burgdorferi* and HIV serology and serum vitamin B_{12} and folate were all normal or negative. Serum immunoglobulins were within the normal range and no paraprotein was seen on serum protein electrophoresis. Antinuclear antibodies and rheumatoid factor were negative. Heavy metal screening including serum lead was negative. Chest X-ray and electrocardiogram were normal on admission. The chest X-ray post-intubation showed signs consistent with aspiration pneumonia. Urine porphyrin screening was negative.

Nerve conduction studies the day after admission were unremarkable apart from delayed or absent F waves, partial motor block from Erb's point and at the fibular head, along with generally low compound muscle action potential amplitudes. Subsequent nerve conduction studies, 3 weeks later, were consistent with a severe, predominantly motor, demyelinating polyneuropathy with associated marked patchy axonal loss.

A diagnostic procedure was performed.

*   *   *

Discussion

If this patient's minor sensory symptoms and signs are first set aside, the differential diagnosis of the clinical presentation becomes that of rapidly progressive lower motor neuron weakness of limb and then bulbar and respiratory muscles (Table 17.1). As soon as the sensory features are included in the analysis, many of these possibilities – specifically diseases of muscle, neuromuscular junction and anterior horn cell – are automatically eliminated, leaving only diseases of peripheral nerves (and/or roots). Similarly, central causes of acute or subacute tetraplegia are readily ruled out. Thus, among other reasons, an acute myelopathy is incompatible with the subsequent development of bulbar palsy. Brainstem encephalitis or infarction would be expected to lead to upper motor neuron features and/or altered consciousness plus more cranial nerve signs.

The remaining major diagnostic category – polyneuropathy – was ultimately supported by the neurophysiological investigations, though the initial electrical findings were relatively mild. Causes of an acute polyneuropathy are summarized in Table 17.2. Again, many may be eliminated on the history and results of investigations. Thus, there was no history of exposure to relevant toxins and heavy metal screening was negative. Lead poisoning is nowadays a rare cause of an acute, predominantly motor, polyneuropathy in adults, usually with a rather different distribution of weakness from this patient (prominent wrist-drop and foot-drop). The patient's serum lead levels were normal. Similarly, an acute motor neuropathy may complicate the hepatic porphyrias, often in association with abdominal pain and CNS features, but this patient's urine porphyrin screen was negative. Vasculitic neuropathy may present acutely but the clinical features are often asymmetrical (multifocal neuropathy – 'mononeuritis multiplex') and this patient had no serological evidence of systemic vasculitis. Critical illness neuropathy develops in patients on an intensive therapy unit with multi-organ failure and is characterized by flaccid weakness and failure to wean from the ventilator.[1] The electro-diagnostic features (as for vasculitic neuropathy) are of an axonal rather than demyelinating neuropathy. There was no clinical or serological

Table 17.1. Differential diagnosis of rapidly progressive lower motor neuron weakness, according to site of lesion.

Muscle
  Hypokalemia
  Rhabdomyolysis
  Polymyositis
Neuromuscular junction
  Myasthenia gravis
  Botulism
Peripheral nerve
  See Table 17.2
Anterior horn cell
  Poliomyelitis

Table 17.2. Causes of acute polyneuropathy.

Guillain–Barré syndrome
Hepatic porphyrias
Toxins, e.g. heavy metals, organophosphates
Vasculitis
Critical illness neuropathy
Meningoradiculopathy secondary to infection, e.g. Lyme disease.
Diphtheria

Table 17.3. Guillain–Barré variants.

Acute inflammatory demyelinating polyneuropathy (classical Guillain–Barré
   syndrome)
Acute motor axonal neuropathy (pure motor variant, no demyelination)
Acute motor sensory axonal neuropathy (fulminant course)
Miller–Fisher syndrome (ophthalmoplegia, ataxia, areflexia)
Acute pandysautonomia (rapid onset autonomic failure)

---

evidence of meningoradiculopathy due to Lyme disease or HIV infection. This leaves only Guillain–Barré syndrome as the likely diagnosis.

   Though there are variants (Table 17.3), classical Guillain–Barré syndrome is defined as a progressive illness with weakness of both legs and arms, and areflexia. Peak deficit must be reached in less than 4 weeks. Motor signs are typically symmetrical and sensory features are mild. Autonomic dysfunction and cranial nerve involvement (bulbar and bifacial palsies) are common, as is back pain. Electrodiagnostic studies in the classical syndrome point to a demyelinating neuropathy – with nerve conduction slowing and/or block – though there may be only minimal electrical abnormalities at onset, as was the case with this patient. Other laboratory features include mildly deranged liver function tests and hyponatremia secondary to inappropriate antidiuretic hormone secretion.

   There is no single diagnostic test for Guillain–Barré syndrome, but the clinical and neurophysiological evidence may be supported by examination of the cerebrospinal fluid. This was therefore the first diagnostic procedure performed on the patient under discussion. The findings are given in Table 17.4 and show the typical elevation of CSF protein with normal white cell count ('dissociation albumino-cytologique'). This was first recognized as an important feature of the syndrome by Guillain, Barré and Strohl in their original description in 1916. In some patients, elevation of the CSF protein may be delayed, or fail to occur at all. Patients with Guillain–Barré syndrome (clinically and electrophysiologi-

Table 17.4. Cerebrospinal fluid findings.

Variable (units)	Finding	Normal range
Appearance	clear, colorless	
Leukocytes (cells/μl)	1	<5
Microorganisms	none	
Culture	negative	
Glucose (mmol/l)	2.8	2.5–3.9
Protein (g/l)	2.6	0.1–0.4

Table 17.5. Organisms associated with Guillain–Barré syndrome.

Campylobacter jejuni
Mycoplasma pneumoniae
Cytomegalovirus (CMV)
Epstein–Barr virus (EBV)
Varicella zoster virus (VZV)
Hepatitis A and B
Human immunodeficiency virus (HIV) 1

cally) but with a CSF pleocytosis are atypical. In the appropriate clinical setting, this combination raises the suspicion of HIV infection.

The etiology of Guillain–Barré syndrome is incompletely understood. An important clue is the observation that there is an antecedent infection in 60–70% of cases. Organisms associated with Guillain–Barré syndrome are listed in Table 17.5. The gastrointestinal illness in this patient's case raised the possibility of *Campylobacter jejuni* infection. This was confirmed by a second diagnostic result: elevated serum antibodies to *Campylobacter jejuni* consistent with recent infection.

The working hypothesis linking antecedent infection with Guillain–Barré syndrome is that the initial illness triggers a process of autoimmune inflammatory demyelination in peripheral nerves. An attractive mechanism for this link is *molecular mimicry*, in which an immune response (both humoral and cell-mediated) is mounted against an infectious organism that shares epitopes with the patient's peripheral nerves. Greater credence may be given to this putative mechanism following immunological studies of the acute motor axonal neuropathy (AMAN) variant of Guillain–Barré syndrome. These studies point to molecules related to ganglioside G_{M1} as the relevant epitopes. Gangliosides are glycolipids which contain sialic acid residues (Fig. 17.1). Their nomenclature was originally devised by Svennerholm. In this system, the subscript letter indicates the number of sialic acid groups. The adjacent numeral is

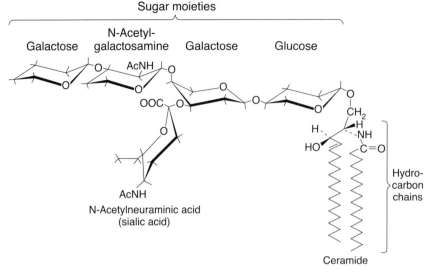

Fig. 17.1. Structure of ganglioside G_{M1}.

$5 - n$, where n is the number of neutral sugar residues. Thus, G_{M1} has one sialic acid group (M = monosialo) and four neutral sugars. G_{M1} and related gangliosides are found in the axolemma of motor nerve fibres.[2] Some *Campylobacter* strains associated with Guillain–Barré syndrome contain G_{M1}-like epitopes in their lipopolysaccharide coats.[3] Anti-G_{M1} antibodies that cross-react with bacterial lipopolysaccharide epitopes are found in Guillain–Barré syndrome patients.[4] Indeed, these antibodies are regularly seen in patients with Guillain–Barré syndrome associated with *Campylobacter jejuni* infection.[5] These strands of evidence all support the notion that bacterial surface molecules excite an antibody response that cross-reacts with shared epitopes on peripheral nerve. The nerve fibers are envisaged as being inadvertently damaged by an immune response origin-ally directed against the infectious agent. The final diagnostic result in the patient under discussion was the detection of high titers of anti-G_{M1} anti-bodies in his serum. It should be noted that other gangliosides are asso-ciated with different variants of Guillain–Barré syndrome. Thus, anti-G_{Q1b} antibodies are commonly seen in Miller–Fisher syndrome.[6] Furthermore, anti-G_{M1} antibodies are not specific for Guillain–Barré syndrome, being found in other neuropathies, notably multifocal motor neuropathy.[7]

Treatment of Guillain–Barré syndrome is twofold: supportive and immunomodulatory. Not all patients progress to the point of requiring ventilatory support. In this patient's case, there were two indications for intubation and ventilation: bulbar dysfunction with risk of aspiration and rapidly deteriorating respiratory function as monitored by the vital capacity. A cut-off value of 1 liter for this variable is usually quoted as indicating a need for assisted ventilation. However, patients who are becoming fatigued with a rapidly deteriorating vital capacity, as was the case with the patient under discussion, should be electively ventilated before this arbitrary level is reached. This patient remained ventilator-dependent for several weeks (a tracheostomy was performed during the first fortnight).

Other supportive measures include monitoring for cardiac arrhythmias and labile blood pressure. Nasogastric feeding should be commenced early, but the autonomic complications of Guillain–Barré syndrome occasionally include a paralytic ileus. Limb weakness warrants regular physiotherapy, to prevent joint stiffness and contractures, and turning, to reduce the risk of pressure sores. Prophylaxis against venous thrombo-embolism includes appropriate stockings and low-dose subcutaneous heparin or equivalent. Mouth and eye care, and aspiration of secretions, should be meticulous. Neuropathic pain may be difficult to treat but sometimes responds to tricyclic antidepressants. Psychological support is important.

Specific immunomodulatory treatments of proven benefit in Guillain–Barré syndrome include plasma exchange and intravenous immunoglobulin.[8] Corticosteroids are ineffective when used in isolation and other immunological approaches remain experimental. Intravenous immunoglobulin is nowadays favored over plasma exchange, because of its ease of administration, and because the trials indicate it is at least as effective.[8] This treatment is reserved for patients whose Guillain–Barré syndrome is sufficiently severe to have rendered them non-ambulant, and who have had symptoms for less than 14 days. The aim of treatment is to increase the rate of recovery and hence reduce the risk of complications.

The prognosis of Guillain–Barré syndrome is adversely affected by several factors including increasing patient age, rapid onset of weakness, need for ventilation, presence of anti-G_{M1} antibodies, preceding diarrheal illness and electrophysiological features showing significant axonal degeneration. Most patients (80%) eventually make a good recovery from a monophasic illness, though this may take many months. Death occurs in 5–10% of patients, due to cardiac arrhythmia, pulmonary embolism or sepsis. More than 10% of patients have permanent disability and a few relapse.

This patient was treated during the first week in hospital with intravenous immunoglobulin (0.4 g/kg daily for five consecutive days) as well as supportive measures. The early aspiration pneumonia responded to intravenous cefotaxime and metronidazole. Though he had several adverse prognostic factors, his muscle power began to improve after several weeks. He was weaned from the ventilator and returned to Canada for further neuro-rehabilitation.

Diagnosis

Guillain–Barré syndrome (acute inflammatory demyelinating polyneuropathy) associated with *Campylobacter jejuni* infection.

References

1. Bolton CF. Critical illness polyneuropathy. In: Asbury AK, Thomas PK, eds. *Peripheral Nerve Disorders* 2. Boston: Butterworth-Heinemann, 1995: 262–280.
2. Corbo M, Quattrini A, Latov N, Hays AP. Localization of GM1 and Gal(β1–3) GalNAc antigenic determinants in peripheral nerve. *Neurology* 1993; **43**: 809–814.
3. Yuki N, Taki T, Inagaki F et al. A bacterium lipopolysaccharide that elicits Guillain–Barré syndrome has a G_{M1} ganglioside-like structure. *J Exp Med* 1993; **178**: 1771–1775.
4. Oomes PG, Jacobs BC, Hazenberg MPH et al. Anti-G_{M1} IgG antibodies and *Campylobacter* bacteria in Guillain–Barré syndrome: evidence of molecular mimicry. *Ann Neurol* 1995; **38**: 170–175.
5. Rees J, Gregson NA, Hughes RAC Anti-ganglioside G_{M1} antibodies in Guillain–Barré syndrome and their relationship to *Campylobacter jejuni* infection. *Ann Neurol* 1995; **38**: 809–816.
6. Chiba A, Kusunoki S, Shimizu T, Kanazawa I. Serum IgG antibody to ganglioside G_{Q1b} is a possible marker of Miller Fisher syndrome. *Ann Neurol* 1992; **31**: 677–679.
7. Pestronk A, Chaudhry V, Feldman EL et al. Lower motor neuron syndromes defined by patterns of weakness, nerve conduction abnormalities and high titers of antiglycolipid antibodies. *Ann Neurol* 1990; **27**: 316–326.
8. van der Meché FGA, Schmitz PIM, the Dutch Guillain–Barré Study Group. A randomized trial comparing intravenous immune globulin and plasma exchange in Guillain–Barré syndrome. *N Engl J Med* 1992; **326**: 1123–1129.

Ataxia in a young girl

Clinical history and examination

HB had an abnormal gait from age 18 months when she began to walk independently. She was later clumsy and unsteady in walking at 4 years.

This girl was born after a full term pregnancy. Her mother had smoked 10 cigarettes a day during the pregnancy but did not take other drugs. The birth weight was 6 pounds 9 ounces (2955 g) and the neonatal period was uneventful. Language and social developmental milestones were normal except for late walking. She did not take independent steps until 18 months and then her gait was unsteady and wide-based. At age 4 years, she was seen by a neurologist when her mother noted progressive worsening of gait, frequent falls and tremulousness during meals. The girl was attending pre-school and performing well except in gross motor skills.

The family history was non-contributory. There were no siblings; the parents were not related.

Physical examination at age 4 years 7 months showed that she was small for age. All growth measures were below the fifth percentile. Otherwise, findings on general examination were unremarkable. There were no dysmorphic features or skin lesions. The fundi and ocular movements were normal. Tendon reflexes were present but depressed. There was mild dysmetria on finger to nose and heel to shin tests. Her gait was broad-based and ataxic. Sensation was probably intact although testing was limited by her age.

MRI of the brain was normal then and again 2 years later (Fig. 18.1a, b, and c). Electrodiagnostic testing showed absence of sensory nerve responses in the legs. Motor nerve conduction velocities were normal and needle EMG was normal. The following blood tests were normal: CBC, CK, LFTs, uric acid, renal function, phytanic acid, B12, folate, vitamin E, lead, porphyrins, thyroid function, lactate, AFP, lipids and immunoglobulins.

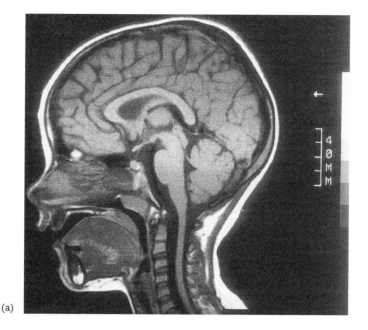

(a)

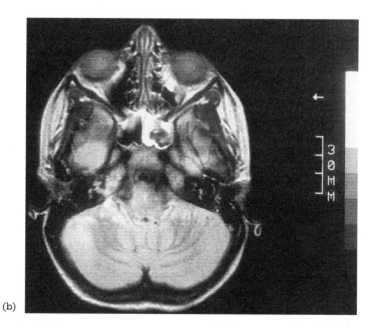

(b)

Fig. 18.1. Magnetic resonance imaging of the brain at age 4 years. (a) Coronal section in midline with normal appearing cerebellum. (b) Axial view shows normal appearing vermis. (c) Axial view of the hemispheres is normal.

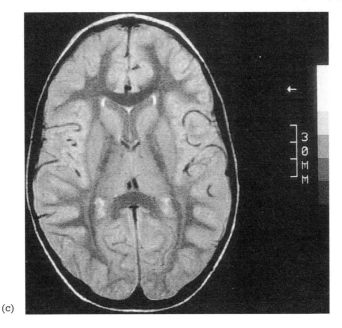

(c)

Fig. 18.1. (*continued*)

At age 5 years, cardiomegaly was seen on chest X-ray and the EKG showed inverted T waves. An echocardiogram revealed left ventricular hypertrophy and an abnormal signal from the papillary muscles. An isotope scan showed normal ventricular function: the ejection fraction was 67%.

Muscle and nerve biopsy were non-diagnostic with only type 1 fiber predominance in the muscle. The nerve biopsy showed depopulation of axons without onion bulbs or ovoids.

By age 5 years 9 months, she could only walk a few steps without support. She used furniture and other objects for support. She complained of pain in her feet and legs. She used a walker for aid. Examination showed mild pes cavus deformity, distal muscle wasting in the legs and a tendency to walk on her toes. Tendon reflexes were absent and vibratory sensation was decreased distally. She was given oral vitamin E supplements.

Over the next year, she developed tight heel cords. Psychometric test results were normal. Ophthalmologic examination was normal. However, the ataxia worsened, nystagmus appeared and position sense was impaired. She had incontinence of urine at school but it was unclear whether this was related to sphincter dysfunction or a mobility problem in getting to the bathroom.

At age 7 years 4 months, she was dysarthric and titubation was seen. A year later, she was wheelchair-dependent. At age 9 years, she was malnourished. The child was placed in foster care while her mother underwent alcohol and drug rehabilitation. Rotary nystagmus was evident and she could not sit without support. A diagnostic test was obtained at age 9 years 6 months.

$$* \quad * \quad *$$

Discussion

This ataxic syndrome was evident at age 18 months. Over the next 5 years motor function deteriorated dramatically. The initial workup was consistent with an axonal neuropathy, perhaps hereditary sensory motor neuropathy type 2, but the family history was negative. Although short stature was noted, the absence of dysmorphic features suggested that this was not a chromosomal disorder or fetal alcohol syndrome. The prominence of limb and truncal ataxia and the presence of a cardiomyopathy indicated that she had a neurodegenerative disease, probably Friedreich ataxia. The differential diagnosis included acquired or hereditary vitamin E deficiency, abetalipoproteinemia, and Refsums disease. Ataxia telangiectasia was also considered but there were no lesions in the conjunctiva. Not until the FRDA gene test was identified could the diagnosis be settled. Mutation analysis in 1997 showed two GAA expanded FRDA alleles of 1050 and 1200 repeats, respectively, confirming the diagnosis of Friedreich ataxia.

Friedreich ataxia is considered the most common hereditary ataxia.[1] It is an autosomal recessive disorder with a variable phenotype. Onset is usually in adolescence and life expectancy is generally about 35 years. In addition to the ataxia, patients show sensory neuropathy, other features are scoliosis, cardiomyopathy, diabetes and dementia. Death generally occurs in the third or fourth decade from heart failure.

The FRDA locus was mapped to 9q13-q21.1 in 1990 where a gene called $X25$ was found.[2] The GAA triplet repeat in this region was reported in 1996.[3] The following year, the protein product, named frataxin, was found to be developmentally regulated and tissue-specific.[4] Genotype–phenotype correlation indicated that the number of repeats correlated with age at onset and severity of symptoms. The phenotypic correlation is with the shorter of the two alleles as this is responsible for producing the residual frataxin; the longer of the two does not seem to matter.[5,6] In our case, the shorter allele had 1050 repeats, predicting a severe phenotype. Symptoms began in late infancy, an unusually early onset. In keeping with the severe phenotype, she had a cardiomyopathy by age 5 years. At age 8 years, she developed scoliosis. Her prognosis is guarded.

Frataxin is localized to the mitochondrial inner membrane and seems to play a role in iron transport within the cell.[7] Strategies for treatment include giving a 'mitochondrial cocktail' that includes vitamins C and K, carnitine, and coenzyme Q to boost mitochondrial function or, perhaps more accurately, to decrease the level of free radicals released in the mitochondria. There is no evidence that this treatment is helpful. Because iron may be accumulating inappropriately within the cell in Friedreich ataxia, some have suggested chelation therapy. However, more study of the function of frataxin and of the role of iron accumulation is needed before such therapy can be recommended.

Diagnosis

Friedreich ataxia.

References

1. Pandolfo M. Molecular pathogenesis of Friedreich ataxia. *Arch Neurol* 1999; **56:** 1201–1208.
2. Shaw J, Lichter P, Driesel AJ, Williamson R, Chamberlain S. Regional localization of the Friedreich ataxia locus to human chromosome 9q13-q21.1. *Cytogenet Cell Genet* 1990; **53:** 221–224.
3. Campuzano V, Montermini L, Molto MD et al. Friedreich ataxia: autosomal recessive disease caused by an intronic GAA triplet repeat expansion. *Science* 1996; **271:** 1423–1427.
4. Duclos F, Boschert U, Sirugo G, Mandel J-L, Hen R, Koenig M. Gene in the region of the Friedreich ataxia locus encodes a putative transmembrane protein expressed in the nervous system. *Proc Natl Acad Sci USA* 1993; **90:** 109–113.
5. Monros E, Molto MD, Martinez F, Canizares J, Blanca J, Vilchez JJ et al. Phenotype correlation and intergenerational dynamics of the Friedreich ataxia GAA trinucleotide repeat. *Am J Hum Genet* 1997; **61:** 101–110.
6. Schols L, Amoiridis G, Przuntek H, Frank G, Epplen JT, Epplen C. Friedreich's ataxia. Revision of the phenotype according to molecular genetics. *Brain* 1997; **120:** 2131–2140.
7. Babcock M, deSilva D, Oaks R, Davis-Kaplan S, Jiralerspong S, Montermini L et al. Regulation of mitochondrial iron accumulation by Yfh1p, a putative homolog of frataxin. *Science* 1997; 276: 1709–1712.

Multiple sclerosis?

Clinical history and examination

In June 1993 at age 28 this woman was in an automobile accident. She suffered a mild concussion with loss of memory for the accident. She then had persistent headaches, neck, and left shoulder pain.

In December 1993 she noted unsteady gait and clumsiness of the left arm. In June 1994, she was found to have dysmetria of the left arm and both legs. The plantar response was up-going on the right and equivocal on the left. Her gait was broad-based and ataxic. She also described emotional lability, anxiety attacks, and cognitive decline.

Brain MRI showed four to five tiny areas of increased signal on T2-weighted images lateral to the margins of the lateral ventricles. There was a vague hyperintensity in the left cerebellar peduncle. WBC was low at 2.4, Hgb was 13.3, HCT 40.5, WSR 4 mm/h, RPR nonreactive, RA screen normal, ANA titer positive at 1:160 (speckled), B12 borderline low at 160 pg/ml, and Lyme EIA normal at 0.15. She was given a diagnosis of multiple sclerosis in July 1994.

In August 1994, i.v. methylprednisolone therapy resulted in a dramatic improvement, but in September 1994 she again noted increasing ataxia, spasticity, and memory problems. Another course of i.v. methylprednisolone resulted in dramatic improvement.

CSF showed an elevated protein at 58 mg %, glucose of 57 mg %, 4 WBC (>90% lymphocytes), VDRL negative, normal IgG index and synthesis rate, negative for oligoclonal bands, and increased myelin basic protein at 1.9 μg/ml. CBC, ACE, HIV titer, HTLV-I titer, and Lyme titer were negative or normal. ANA remained elevated at 1:640, rheumatoid factor was increased to 26, but anti-DNA, ENA, and SS-A were negative. Anti-Hu antibody was negative. PPD was negative and CXR was normal. Serum protein electrophoresis showed polyclonal hypergammaglobulinemia. Repeat MRI showed multiple areas of abnormal T2 hyperintensity in the white matter (Fig. 19.1), with innumerable punctate areas of

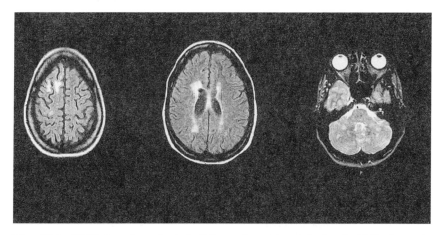

Fig. 19.1. Multiple subcortical (left image), periventricular (middle image), and brainstem (right image) T2 hyperintense lesions.

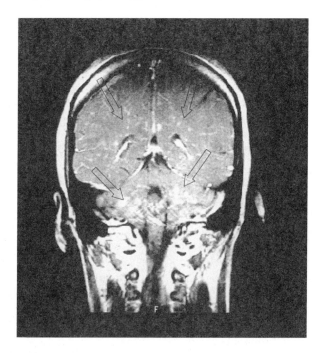

Fig. 19.2. Gadolinium enhancement of multiple small lesions evident on a coronal image from the MRI study of Fig. 19.1.

enhancement after gadolinium administration (Fig. 19.2). A cerebral angiogram was normal, with no evidence of vasculitis.

She again worsened in October 1994. A third course of i.v. methylprednisolone was accompanied by transient improvement. In December 1994 she was given weekly oral doses of methotrexate. In January 1995 she developed increased confusion and ataxia. She was again treated with i.v. methylprednisolone, but with transient improvement. On March 16, 1995 a right temporal lobe tip biopsy was performed.

*   *   *

Discussion

Tissue from the right partial temporal lobectomy showed prominent, perivascular-based chronic inflammation consisting primarily of lymphocytic cells (Fig. 19.3).

Although the white matter was more severely involved, there was also focal involvement of gray matter. In areas, the lymphoid infiltrate became somewhat confluent. Intervening reactive astrocytes were prominently noted. Macrophages were not prominently seen. Scattered lymphoid cells showed marked nuclear enlargement and coarse chromatin pattern, and irregularities to the nuclear contour (Fig. 19.4).

The cells stained positively for CD20 (B-cell lymphoid marker). Most lymphoid cells, however, stained positively for CD3 (T-cell lymphoid marker) and had the morphology of reactive lymphocytes. The histologic appearance of the lesion was most consistent with a malignant non-Hodgkin lymphoma, large cell type (B-cell immunophenotype) (REAL

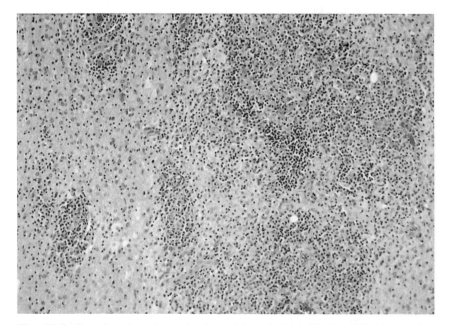

Fig. 19.3. Prominent perivascular-based lymphoid infiltrate with intervening gliotic white matter. (Hematoxylin and eosin, original magnification 100×)

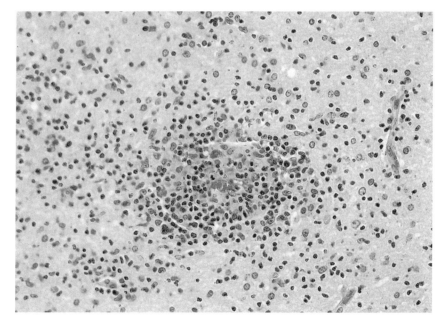

Fig. 19.4. Scattered atypical-appearing, perivascular, lymphoid cells consistent with lymphoma. (Hematoxylin and eosin, original magnification 400×)

classification) with prominent numbers of tumor-infiltrating lymphocytes. She was treated with high dose i.v. methotrexate and intrathecal methotrexate, followed by whole brain radiotherapy to 4000 cGy with a 1440 cGy boost. This was followed by two cycles of intravenous ARA-C.

Although much of the pathology was white matter based, raising inflammatory demyelinating disease as a differential diagnostic consideration, a few features suggested otherwise. Focal involvement of gray matter by inflammation is generally absent in most inflammatory demyelinating conditions. Although the presence of a perivascular-based chronic inflammatory cell infiltrate and reactive astrocytosis may be consistent with a demyelinating lesion, the paucity of white matter macrophages and lack of evidence of myelin loss suggested some other condition.

Particularly salient in this case were the presence of lymphoid cells with atypical cytologic features: nuclear enlargement, irregularities in nuclear contour and a coarse chromatin pattern. Immunohistochemistry demonstrated that the atypical lymphoid cells had a B-cell immunophenotype, in contrast to the bulk of the other smaller, benign appearing lymphoid cells which were noted to have a T-cell immunophenotype. Morphologically, these features were consistent with a large cell lymphoma, including a prominent component of benign tumor-infiltrating lymphocytes (TIL). TIL infiltrates are common in primary CNS lymphomas. Confirmation of diagnosis, particularly in cases where cytologic atypia is not readily evident or is obscured by a prominent TIL component can be obtained by ancillary molecular biologic techniques such as gene rearrangement.

This patient was initially given a diagnosis of MS, based on relapses and remission, along with multicentric white matter lesions, and improvement after intravenous methylprednisolone treatment. She exhibited atypical MRI features, consisting of an unusual pattern of gadolinium enhancement. She had miliary focal enhancement, and all lesions appeared similar after gadolinium administration. This pattern is distinctly unusual in MS, where only a proportion of lesions show enhancement.

Primary central nervous system lymphoma[1,2] accounts for approximately 1% of all intracranial neoplasms. It is observed in patients with immunodeficiency syndromes, such as AIDS, but may be seen in patients without obvious immunocompromise, as in the current case. Also, as in this case, primary CNS lymphoma may include multiple lesions, and can be confused with metastatic disease, sarcoidosis, or MS.[3] Primary CNS lymphoma may respond favorably, although transiently, to treatment with corticosteroids.[4]

The manifestations of primary CNS lymphoma are similar in immunocompromised and immunocompetent people. The patient may show signs of an intracranial mass lesion, mental status changes, or focal neurologic signs. In 40% of cases, primary CNS lymphoma shows multiple lesions in the brain. Behavioral and mental status changes occur in the majority of patients. Most commonly, MRI shows a single or multiple enhancing parenchymal lesions. The multiple persistently enhancing lesions were considered atypical for MS in this case and led to a brain biopsy. Cerebrospinal fluid pleocytosis and higher protein content were consistent with primary CNS lymphoma. Cytologic examination of the cells may identify the malignancy, but a predominance of reactive T lymphocytes (see biopsy) in CSF may obscure the underlying diagnosis.

Diagnosis

CNS lymphoma.

References

1. Koeller KK, Smirniotopoulos JG, Jones RV. Primary central nervous system lymphoma: radiologic–pathologic correlation. (Review). *Radiographics* 1997; **17**: 1497–1526.
2. Johnson BA, Fram EK, Johnson PC, Jacobowitz R. The variable MR appearance of primary lymphoma of the central nervous system: comparison with histopathologic features. *Am J Neuroradiol* 1997; **18**: 563–572.
3. DeAngelis LM. Primary central nervous system lymphoma imitates multiple sclerosis. *J Neuro-Oncol* 1990; **9**: 177–181.
4. Singh A, Strobos RJ, Singh BM, Rothballer AB, Reddy V, Puljic S et al. Steroid-induced remissions in CNS lymphoma. *Neurology* 1982; **32**: 1267–1271.

20

Diplopia and ptosis in a young man

Clinical history and examination

A 27-year-old man was seen at the Neuro-ophthalmology Outpatient Clinic having been referred from a neighboring hospital.

He had been attending the ophthalmology department of that hospital for just over 1 year with mild horizontal diplopia for which his glasses had been fitted with corrective prisms, and a presumptive diagnosis of decompensated exophoria had been made.

Three months ago whilst watching television he had experienced double vision different to his previous diplopia, with vertical separation of images, worse on upgaze, which had persisted. He recalled that about 2 months prior to the onset of these symptoms he had knocked the right side of his head against a kitchen unit, which whilst acutely painful had not been associated with any disturbance of consciousness or other symptoms. On direct questioning, he had found that his symptoms seemed worse when he was particularly tired but, in general, there had not been a consistent pattern of diurnal variation or fluctuation. In the past week he had noticed in the mirror that the eyelid of his right eye had begun to droop and also felt that vision in that eye had deteriorated rapidly over the past 4 days.

A resident in the UK since the age of 12, he had been born in Sierra Leone, to which he had returned briefly on four occasions, the last 7 months previously. He was a non-smoker and did not take alcohol. Five years ago he had been successfully treated for Hodgkins lymphoma with chemotherapy and thoracic radiotherapy and at follow-up to date there had been no evidence of recurrence. His older brother had been treated 2 years ago for suspected pulmonary tuberculosis. There was no other personal or family history of significant illness including diabetes mellitus or thyroid disease.

On examination he had a right subtotal ptosis. Manual elevation of the right upper eyelid revealed that the right eye was depressed in the primary position. The cover test demonstrated that, of the two images he saw, the upper image originated from the right eye. The pupils were 2 mm at rest and reacted symmetrically to light and on convergence. Bilaterally visual acuity was 6/9 correcting to 6/6 with pinhole and visual fields were normal to confrontation and on static (Humphrey) perimetry. No errors were made on Ishihara isochromatic plate testing. There were no abnormal fundoscopic findings. Pursuit and saccadic eye movements in the left eye were normal. He was unable to elevate the right eye fully, a finding present in both the primary position and in abduction and adduction. Downward and lateral ductions were normal. The pattern of ophthalmoparesis was the same during testing of the vestibulo-ocular reflex (the doll's head maneuver).

Prolonged upgaze did not exacerbate the degree of ptosis on the right nor reveal ptosis on the left. Testing of the rest of the cranial nerves was normal except for relative weakness of orbicularis oculi bilaterally. Strength in head extensors and proximal limb musculature was normal, as was the rest of the neurological examination, including gait and coordination. There was no evidence of jaundice, anemia or lymphadenopathy. Examination of the chest and abdomen was normal.

In this patient the FBC, blood film, ESR and CRP and fasting glucose were all within normal limits. ANA, ANCA and VDRL were negative. Magnetic resonance imaging of the brain, with and without gadolinium enhancement, were within normal limits, as were fat-suppressed images of the orbits. Cerebrospinal fluid examination was also unremarkable. A diagnostic test was performed.

*   *   *

Discussion

The combination of unilateral partial ptosis and extraocular muscle dysfunction may suggest a partial oculomotor nerve (third cranial nerve) palsy, where the muscle involved is other than the lateral rectus and superior oblique muscles. The finding in this case that only elevation was involved and that this was evident in both the adducted and abducted position suggests dysfunction of both superior rectus and inferior oblique muscles, a so-called 'double elevator' palsy.

First, we will review the consequences of lesions at various stages in the anatomical course of the third cranial nerve and then discuss how the clinical picture of a double elevator palsy with ptosis might arise.

Each oculomotor nerve supplies the ipsilateral eye. In theory, the site of a neural lesion causing an oculomotor nerve palsy could be supranuclear, nuclear or infranuclear.[1] At each level, possible lesion etiologies include vascular, neoplastic, inflammatory and infectious.

Supranuclear lesions are occasionally seen and may result from pre-motor lesions either local to the oculomotor nuclear complex in the midbrain or at more disparate sites. They are distinguished from nuclear lesions by preservation of oculomotor nerve function during vestibulo-ocular or caloric testing.

Because the cell bodies of both oculomotor nerves lie in close proximity within the oculomotor nuclear complex, nuclear lesions tend to produce bilateral oculomotor nerve dysfunction. Bilateral symmetrical ptosis may or may not be present depending upon whether or not there is involvement of the single midline central caudal nucleus (CCN), which innervates both levator palpebrae superiori. Fibers supplying superior rectus originate from a specific subnucleus within the contralateral part of the oculomotor nucleus complex. Since they decussate through the equivalent ipsilateral subnucleus, lesions of the oculomotor nucleus complex which are discrete enough to be unilateral invariably produce a contralateral palsy of superior rectus accompanying a complete ipsilateral third nerve palsy. Nuclear third nerve lesions may be pupil-sparing. When present, pupillary involvement indicates that the dorsal, rostral part of the oculo-motor nuclear complex is involved in the lesion, usually bilaterally. Smaller lesions, damaging a focal part or parts of the oculomotor nuclear complex, may selectively affect innervation of any one or more of the extra-ocular muscles supplied by the third nerve.[1]

Within the midbrain or rostral pons, an infranuclear deficit may be produced by damage to the individual fascicles contributing to the oculo-motor nerve, or to the entire nerve itself before it emerges into the sub-arachnoid space. It is now established, largely through clinical correlation with high-resolution MR imaging,[2–4] that involvement of one or more of these fascicles can mimic any pattern of palsy of muscles supplied by the oculomotor nerve, usually, though not always, with concurrent pupil dila-tation.

The same lesion types may be responsible for supranuclear, nuclear or infranuclear lesions intrinsic to the midbrain. Most are vascular and due to occlusion of, or hemorrhage from, perforating branches of the basilar or posterior cerebral arteries or, less commonly, complete occlusion of the distal part of the basilar artery ('top of the basilar syndrome'). Where discrete vascular areas are involved, classical clinical pictures are described, such as the oculomotor nerve palsy and contralateral involun-tary movements of Benedikts syndrome due to infarction of the nerve, or its fascicles, as they pass through the dorsocaudal aspect of the red nucleus. Webers syndrome, consisting of an oculomotor nerve palsy and paresis of contralateral face and body, is due to midbrain infarction ventral to the red nucleus, though the same clinical syndrome may arise from mass lesions compressing the ventral surface of the midbrain. Of the neoplastic lesions, the commonest primary tumors are gliomas. Secondary deposits from, for example, breast, lung, and prostate become more likely with increasing age. Demyelinating lesions of multiple sclerosis or post-infectious inflammation are also commonly seen. Other intrinsic lesions include the inflammatory lesions of granulomatous conditions such as neurosarcoidosis.

At any stage, from the point of its emergence from the midbrain into the interpeduncular fossa, its piercing of the dura to enter the cavernous sinus, and up to the point at which it enters the orbit through the superior orbital fissure, the oculomotor nerve is vulnerable to compression from aneurysms of either the basilar, posterior cerebral, or internal carotid arteries, but most commonly the posterior communicating artery. Other examples of compressive pathology include extrinsic tumor such as a meningioma of the sphenoid wing or a nasopharyngeal carcinoma, a hematoma or abscess, and pressing of the nerve against the free edge of the tentorium by the hippocampal gyrus of the temporal lobe during uncal herniation. The nerve may also be compressed within the cavernous sinus by aneurysmal dilatation of the internal carotid artery or a caroticocavernous fistula. In most cases compressive lesions are not pupil-sparing but rather result early-on in a fixed, dilated pupil because of the superficial position of the pupillomotor fibers in the nerve.

Other pathologies extrinsic to the brainstem include acute and chronic infectious meningitis, malignant meningitis and meningovascular syphilis.

Oculomotor palsy after severe trauma, when not the result of uncal herniation, is common and probably represents traction or contusion of the nerve at various points in its course. Onset at a delayed interval following minor trauma is also described, but rare.

Occlusive disease of the vasa nervorum causing infarction of the nerve is the commonest cause of a pupil-sparing oculomotor nerve palsy. Preservation of pupillary function probably reflects better collateral supply to the more superficial part of the nerve which contains the pupil-lomotor fibers. The commonest risk factors occurring in the elderly are diabetes mellitus, systemic hypertension and a history of ischemic heart disease, and most cases resolve within about 6 months. Sometimes vascular compromise of the nerve is accompanied by internal ophthalmo-plegia and this, taken together with the common symptom of periorbital pain at the time of onset, which can be severe, means that neuroimaging may be needed to exclude an expanding or ruptured aneurysm. Systemic vasculitides such as giant cell arteritis, polyarteritis nodosa and systemic lupus erythematosus may also give rise to the same clinical presentation.

Oculomotor neuropathy may also be a consequence of Guillain–Barré syndrome, may follow infection with Epstein–Barr virus or mycoplasma, or may occur in the context of serum gammopathies or systemic or primary cerebral lymphoma, such as occurs in AIDS.

Although cases are reported of oculomotor nerve palsy as a sole mani-festation, lesions involving the nerve as it passes through the cavernous sinus or superior orbital fissure tend, variously, to also affect the adjacent trochlear, abducens and optic nerves. In addition to compression from aneurysms, compression may occur from local primary tumors such as meningioma, craniopharyngioma and pituitary tumors, infiltrating naso-pharyngioma or metastatic carcinoma or lymphoma. The condition of idiopathic granulomatous pseudotumour (Tolosa–Hunt syndrome) has a predilection for the region of the orbital apex stretching back through the superior orbital fissure into the cavernous sinus. The usual presentation is with periorbital pain, oculomotor or visual deficit, depending upon which nerves are involved, and, variably, proptosis. The pseudotumor is usually visible on MRI though its radiological appearances are not diagnostic of the lesion. Response to systemic steroids is often rapid and complete but relapse, once steroids are tapered, is a frequent management problem.

As it enters the orbit, the oculomotor nerve divides into a superior division, which innervates the levator palpebrae and superior rectus muscles, and an inferior division, which carries pupillomotor fibers (via the ciliary ganglion) and innervates the remainder of the extraocular muscles supplied by the oculomotor nerve. Isolated superior or inferior branch palsies due to intraocular pathology are well described but, because of the ability of more proximal lesions to mimic the clinical signs of these syndromes, localization on clinical criteria cannot be presumed.

Finally, disease of the neuromuscular junction, the commonest adult acquired form being myasthenia gravis, should be considered in any case of pupil-sparing ophthalmoparesis, especially that accompanied with ptosis.[5]

Other causes of ptosis include unilateral congenital ptosis, Horners syndrome, myotonic dystrophy, ocular dystrophies and mitochondrial cytopathy; none of which were relevant to this case.

Opinions differ over the localization of lesions leading to apparent 'double elevator' palsies, both those seen as a congenital defect in children and as an acquired deficit in adulthood. When elevation during VOR testing is preserved a supranuclear lesion is presumed.[6] Nuclear deficits in apparent monocular palsy of the elevator muscles are unlikely since the innervation of superior rectus is crossed, but that of inferior oblique is not. Cases of selective damage to the fascicles carrying fibers to superior rectus and inferior oblique muscles are documented. Since these muscles are innervated by fibers which diverge in the orbit into separate branches of the oculomotor nerve, this clinical picture is unlikely to result from a lesion at the orbital level. However, it must be emphasized that neural lesions causing elevator palsy, as described above, are rare and by far the commonest causes of this picture is indeed due to orbital disease, namely diseases which physically restrict elevation of the globe, like Graves' ophthalmopathy or traumatic orbital fracture, or reduce the efficacy of neuromuscular transmission, like myasthenia gravis.

Investigation

Simple investigations of an isolated oculomotor nerve palsy in a previously well adult should be directed towards screening for the commoner and more easily diagnosable causes. The full blood count (FBC) and blood film may directly reveal a proliferative disorder of myeloid or lymphoid origin or may show evidence of immunosuppression or response to infection. Elevation of the erythrocyte sedimentation rate or C-reactive protein may be a general indicator of inflammation, infection or neoplastic disease or may be specifically helpful in the diagnosis of giant cell arteritis in the appropriate clinical context. A fasting glucose should be performed and the systemic blood pressure reading taken. A clotting screen may point towards an underlying thrombotic tendency. Testing for antinuclear antibodies (ANA) and antinucleolar cytoplasmic antibody (ANCA) as an indicator of vasculitis, and a VDRL, looking for evidence of previous syphilis infection, should be performed.

Except where the clinical picture strongly suggests an uncomplicated pupil-sparing oculomotor palsy of vascular origin in, for example, an elderly diabetic or hypertensive patient, and monthly review shows no deterioration, neuroimaging to exclude a compressive or mass lesion is always indicated. Computed tomography provides a useful screening tool for a mass lesion or an aneurysm larger than 1 cm but is not sensitive enough to detect focal lesions, especially in the brainstem or the orbits, which requires MR imaging. If the diagnosis is still not apparent the cerebrospinal fluid (CSF) should be examined looking for cellular changes consistent with infection or inflammation, for changes in the protein level suggestive of an inflammatory polyneuropathy or post-infectious demyelination, for oligoclonal bands and for the presence of malignant cells. Blood and CSF serological testing for Epstein–Barr virus and mycoplasma may also be warranted. A chest X-ray and serum angiotensin-converting enzyme (ACE) level may detect underlying sarcoidosis.

Ptosis of this patient's right eyelid had been almost complete from the initial examination and it had not been possible to demonstrate eyelid fatigue clinically. There was no evidence of fatiguability in any of the other muscle groups although strength of orbicularis oculi was mildly impaired. However, since the patient himself had felt that his symptoms had been slowly worsening and showed minimal fluctuation, he was admitted for a Tensilon test (Fig. 20.1). Using the degree of ptosis at rest as an objective measure of weakness, the Tensilon test proved positive, with maximal voluntary separation of the right eyelids increasing from 2 to 6 mm after 10 mg of intravenous edrophonium, confirming a diagnosis of myasthenia gravis with predominant ocular involvement. Because of this positive diagnostic result a forced-duction test was not performed, though this may be a valuable test in identifying ophthalmoplegia due to restrictive intraorbital disease.

Further discussion

Myasthenia gravis is an autoimmune neurological disease characterized

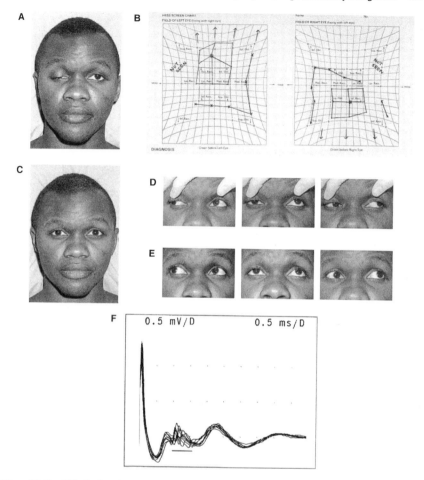

Fig. 20.1. (A) Patient's appearance before the edrophonium (Tensilon) test. (B) Hess chart before treatment (positions for each eye when viewing target positions with fellow eye under conditions of ocular dissociation) showing underaction of superior rectus and inferior oblique in the right eye with compensatory overaction on the other side, according to Herings Law. (C) Appearance after 10 mg edrophonium. (D) Vertical gaze positions (up-to-the-left, directly up, up-and-to-the-right) before edrophonium. (E) Vertical gaze positions after 10 mg edrophonium. (F) Single-fiber EMG recording from right orbicularis oculi muscle showing increased dispersion of motor unit response latencies known as 'jitter' (–) characteristic of myasthenia gravis.

clinically by muscle weakness and fatiguability and is due to T cell-dependent B cell production of polyclonal and heterogeneous antibodies directed against acetylcholine (ACh) receptors. These antibodies decrease the number of functional post-synaptic ACh receptors at the motor end plate to about one-third of normal by directly sterically blocking the receptor's active site, by inducing complement-mediated damage of the post-synaptic membrane, and by also increasing the rate of endocytosis and degradative turnover of the receptor. Whilst the normal decrement in ACh release at the neuromuscular junction which occurs with repetitive muscle activity does not affect the efficacy of neurotransmission, in patients with myasthenia gravis depletion of the functional reserve of ACh receptors means that diminishing ACh release is associated with increasing transmission failure. This mechanism is directly responsible for the clinical phenomenon of muscle fatiguability in myasthenia gravis.

Anti-ACh receptor antibodies are probably present in all acquired myasthenia gravis but are only detected with current assays in between 80 and 90% of patients. Overall, antibody levels are not useful in determining disease severity between patients but can be used to monitor the clinical course for the same patient: relapses being associated with a rise in the titre and remission with a fall.

Myasthenia gravis affects all races and all ages, peaking in incidence in young women and older males. Characteristically onset of muscle weakness is insidious and highly variable from day to day and week to week, often worsening as the day progresses. Ninety per cent with the disease will at some time have involvement of levator palpebrae superioris or the extraocular muscles, and in 70% it is present at presentation.

In some patients, symptoms remain predominantly ocular and for such patients the term 'ocular myasthenia' is commonly used. However, it must be stressed that this group have the same disease, that subclinical generalized muscle involvement can be demonstrated electrophysiologically, and that, usually within 2 years of presentation, a significant number will go on to develop symptomatic generalized weakness. Ptosis is a common presenting sign, sometimes associated with contralateral overaction of frontalis muscle. It is often unilateral and may move from eye to eye but eventually becomes bilateral in most patients. A feature of the examination is that ptosis is exacerbated by prolonged upgaze. Rapid recovery, then fatigue, of levator palpebrae superioris leads to the occasional observation of twitching of a drooping eyelid upon upgaze after a period of rest during downgaze (Cogans lid twitch sign).

When the extraocular muscles are involved there is usually some degree of accompanying ptosis. Myasthenia is 'the great impersonator' and extraocular muscle involvement can mimic any ocular nerve palsy, internuclear ophthalmoplegia or gaze palsy, in isolation or varied combination, or may produce an ophthalmoparesis which does not conform to conventional patterns of ocular neuromuscular deficit. Fatigue of accommodation may also lead to a patient complaining of 'blurring' of near vision only.

Both intrasaccadic and intersaccadic fatigue may be evident in any aspect of the trajectory, velocity and amplitude of patient's saccadic eye movements. Whilst large saccades are often hypometric, small saccades may be hypermetric, probably as a consequence of central upregulation of the saccadic pulse. Mid-saccade slowing may also result in apparent sliding of the eye into its final position. Fatigue of tonic fibers means that gaze position is poorly held and the eye tends to drift back at the end of a saccade. Various patterns of gaze-evoked nystagmus may be observed.

As part of the examination of a patient with ptosis and/or ophthalmoparesis, the strength of orbicularis oculi should be specifically tested. If weakness is present, this finding supports a diagnosis of myasthenia gravis as a potential cause of accompanying ocular signs. Whilst it is debatable whether or not pupillary function is involved, it is hardly ever clinically apparent. The commonest sites of systemic involvement are the neck extensors and proximal limb muscles and these should be specifically tested for weakness and fatiguability. The muscles of deglutition and phonation are also commonly affected. If bulbar or respiratory function is compromised the condition may become rapidly life-threatening ('myasthenic crisis'), an emergency which is seen more often in the elderly.

The most useful diagnostic investigation is the Tensilon (edrophonium) test. Before performing the test, it is crucial to identify a measure which can be used as objective evidence of clinical improvement. Commonly this is the time taken for ptosis to supervene on prolonged upgaze, or the measured size of the palpebral fissure. If diplopia is the predominant symptom, red–green spectacles can be used so that the patient can report any improvement in the separation of true and false visual images, but this is open to patient bias. Interestingly, where the size of an eso- or exo-tropia can be judged to have improved by the examiner, patients are frequently subjectively oblivious to the improvement.

The Tensilon test should only be performed in the presence of a doctor qualified in techniques of basic life support and standard resuscitation facilities should be immediately at hand. Patients with a history of serious heart disease are not suitable for the test. Patients should be forewarned of the usually minor side-effects that accompany the test. Ideally a placebo condition should be employed and the operator and patient blinded to the order in which drug and placebo tests are given. First a dose of 2 mg of edrophonium is injected and the patient assessed over the next 2 minutes. If there is no sign of improvement then the remainder of the total dose of 10 mg is given. Excessive cholinergic side-effects may be countered by co-administration of atropine. If there is still no sign of benefit after 3 minutes the test is negative. A negative test does in itself not preclude a diagnosis of myasthenia gravis. Repeating the test on several occasions may eventually be rewarded by a conclusively positive test, especially when the patient's symptoms are at their worst. Where a patient's general health contraindicates a Tensilon test, transient amelioration of ocular signs by the 2 minute application of an ice-filled surgical glove to the most affected eye (the ice test) may be a useful alternative indicator of the diagnosis.

Supportive investigations include the detection of anti-ACh receptor antibodies in the patient's serum, which are highly specific for the disease but are present in only about 50% of patients who have predominantly the eye signs of the disease.[7] In an experienced operator's hands, the detection of conduction block and increased variability of latencies between nerve fiber activation and muscle fiber action potential (known as 'jitter') during single fiber electromyography has also been shown to be a sensitive investigation for the diagnosis of myasthenia gravis.[8] In predominantly ocular myasthenia gravis, frontalis is the muscle examined.

Once the diagnosis is confirmed, an important ancillary investigation is either CT or MR imaging of the thorax to detect thymoma, which is present in 10% of patients and can be malignant. Since myasthenia gravis patients have an increased incidence of all autoimmune diseases, it may be useful to screen for at least some of these, particularly for diabetes and thyroid disease, but this will in part be directed by the personal and family history and the results of baseline investigations. Physicians should always be aware of the possibility of coexistence of thyroid ophthalmopathy and ocular myasthenia gravis.

Initial therapy consists of an anticholinesterase agent such as pyridostigmine. In our experience, however, patients with predominantly ocular myasthenia hardly ever receive significant benefit from these drugs. In those requiring treatment, the mainstay remains alternate day systemic corticosteroids. An introductory dose of 10 mg is usually sufficient for improvement and if not may be gradually increased until the patient's symptoms are significantly and stably improved. After 3 months, attempts should be made in small dose steps to move towards an alternate day regimen.

Identification of patients at risk of serious side-effects of long-term steroids, in particular insulin resistance and osteoporosis, must be actively anticipated and treated.

Slow tapering of the total steroid dose should not be considered until a stable response has been established, which usually takes about 6 months to 1 year. Inappropriately precipitate tapering is very likely to result in relapse, often at a delayed interval.

Thymectomy may be a useful therapy particularly in patients under 50 years of age with systemic symptoms of myasthenia gravis not controlled adequately by anticholinesterases. It is usual to delay giving steroids to these patients until weeks after the operation and sometimes necessary to institute a course of plasmapheresis pre-operatively to maximize fitness for surgery.

Azathioprine[9] and cyclosporin[10] represent alternative immunosuppressive agents of proven value. The onset of action of azathioprine is slower than steroids and so is initially given as an adjunct for about 6 months to 1 year before consideration is given to reduction in the steroid dose. Full blood count and liver function tests need monitoring regularly and doses adjusted accordingly.

With its protean manifestations, myasthenia gravis should always be considered in any case of localized or generalized muscular weakness, since it is treatable and failure to recognize the condition can lead to substantial morbidity and occasionally mortality. Where the extraocular muscles are involved, it can mimic almost any presentation of latent or manifest strabismus, internuclear ophthalmoplegia or paresis of gaze.

Diagnosis

Myasthenia gravis.

References

1. Smith, CH. Nuclear and infranuclear ocular motility disorders. In: Miller N, Newman N, editors. *Walsh & Hoyt's Clinical Neuro-Ophthalmology.* 5th edn. Baltimore: Williams & Wilkins, 1998; 1189–1281.
2. Hriso E, Masdeu JC, Miller A. Monocular elevation weakness and ptosis – an oculomotor fascicular syndrome. *Journal of Clinical Neuro-Ophthalmology* 1991; **11:** 111–113.
3. Ksiazek SM, Slamovits TL, Rosen CE, Burde RM, Parisi F. Fascicular arrangement in partial oculomotor paresis. *American Journal of Ophthalmology* 1994; **118:** 97–103.
4. Schwartz TH, Lycette CA, Yoon SS, Kargman DE. Clinicoradiographic evidence for oculomotor fascicular anatomy. *Journal of Neurology Neurosurgery and Psychiatry* 1995; **59:** 338.
5. Kuncl R, Hoffman P. Myopathies and disorders of neuromuscular transmission. In: Miller N, Newman N, editors. *Walsh & Hoyt's Clinical Neuro-Ophthalmology.* 5th edn. Baltimore: Williams & Wilkins, 1998; 1351–1460.
6. Zee D. Supranuclear and internuclear ocular motor disorders. In: Miller N, Newman N, editors. *Walsh & Hoyt's Clinical Neuro-Ophthalmology.* 5th edn. Baltimore: Williams & Wilkins, 1998; 1283–1349.
7. Vincent A, Newsom-Davis J. Acetylcholine-receptor antibody as a diagnostic-test for myasthenia-gravis – results in 153 validated cases and 2967 diagnostic assays. *Journal of Neurology, Neurosurgery and Psychiatry* 1985; **48:** 1246–1252.
8. Sanders DB. The electrodiagnosis of myasthenia-gravis. *Annals of the New York Academy of Sciences* 1987; **505:** 539–556.
9. Mantegazza R, Antozzi C, Peluchetti D, Sghirlanzoni A, Cornelio F. Azathioprine as a single drug or in combination with steroids in the treatment of myasthenia-gravis. *Journal of Neurology* 1988; **235:** 449–453.
10. Tindall RSA, Rollins JA, Phillips JT, Greenlee RG, Wells L, Belendiuk G. Preliminary results of a double-blind, randomized, placebo-controlled trial of cyclosporine myasthenia-gravis. *New England Journal of Medicine* 1987; **316:** 719–724.

Young onset stroke

A 40-year-old man presented to the Emergency Department with rapid onset of impaired vision. He had noticed loss of vision to the left 6 hours previously and had been bumping into objects, was unable to see complete faces and had difficulty reading. His speech was normal.

He had no headache or neck ache and there was no history of recent trauma. Limb function was normal. There was no past medical history of relevance other than occasional attacks of migraine with aura. However, they were infrequent and he had not had any for 8 months. Both parents were alive. His mother aged 67 suffered from non-insulin dependent diabetes mellitus. His father aged 68 had suffered a myocardial infarct the year before. He had no siblings. He worked as a storekeeper, smoked 20 cigarettes per day, drank 1 unit of alcohol per day and took neither prescribed nor recreational drugs. He was heterosexual with no recognized risk of HIV exposure.

Examination found him to be mildly drowsy but orientated. Blood pressure was 140/85, temperature 37.2°C. Speech was normal in content and articulation. He had a left homonymous hemianopia. The remainder of the cranial nerves and neurological examination were normal. General examination was also unremarkable; in particular he was in sinus rhythm with normal heart sounds and no carotid bruits.

Full blood count, electrolytes, liver function tests and random glucose were normal. His ESR was 36. A pro-coagulation screen including levels of protein S, C and anti-thrombin III was normal. An electrocardiogram was within normal limits and his chest X-ray clear. Computed tomography (CT) scanning demonstrated some low density changes in the right parieto-occipital region.

The patient was admitted. His hemianopia resolved by 48 hours after his presentation to hospital, and his conscious level returned to normal. Additional investigations showed normal fasting lipids and echocardiogram and a negative autoimmune profile including tests for anti-phospholipid antibodies. Serological tests for syphilis were also negative. Carotid Doppler ultrasonography did not identify any significant stenosis.

The patient was discharged on aspirin 300 mg daily. When seen in clinic 8 weeks later he was well and had returned to work.

Seven months after his original presentation he was transferred to a neurological service as an emergency with acute onset of right-sided paralysis. On arrival he was apyrexial but drowsy and confused. There was no papilledema but he did have a right homonymous hemianopia. He had a moderate dysphasia and a severe (MRC grade 3) weakness of his right upper and lower limbs with an upper motor neuron pattern of right facial weakness.

General examination was normal. Blood pressure was 130/90.

Standard hematological and biochemical blood studies and peripheral inflammatory markers were within normal limits. An MRI scan showed evidence of ischemic changes affecting both parieto-occipital lobes in addition to further ischemic changes involving the left temporo-parietal region. An MR angiogram was normal.

The patient's conscious state improved but his weakness persisted. A diagnostic procedure was performed.

*   *   *

Discussion

This man's first presentation was as a young-onset stroke – for which there is a standard, albeit ever increasing, list for differential diagnosis.

The CT scan excluded any hemorrhagic cause for the hemianopia and likewise the MRI did not demonstrate hemorrhage as the cause of the hemiparesis. Clinical examination, ECG and echocardiography helped to exclude a cardiac source of embolization. At present there is debate as to whether a transesophageal echocardiogram (TOE) should be undertaken in such patients even if the 2-D transthoracic ECHO is normal. A TOE would have unequivocally excluded an atrial source of embolus. The carotid Dopplers, and subsequently the MR angiogram, demonstrated satisfactory blood flow in the carotids and vertebral arteries and specifically no area of significant stenosis. However, given the location of the first stroke, a vertebral artery dissection should have entered the differential diagnosis in this man,[1] despite the absence of neck pain or headache in the acute episode. MR angiography should have been performed at the patient's first presentation. Treatment of an acute dissection with heparin then warfarin anticoagulation has been shown to reduce the risk of extending strokes without significantly increasing intracranial hemorrhage frequency.

Additional causes of young onset stroke include the arteritides. However, this patient has no clinical, immunological or radiological evidence of widespread vasculitis. Disorders affecting blood vessel structure e.g. Ehlers–Danlos syndrome, Moya Moya disease are usually apparent either on clinical examination or arterial angiography – as would the inflammatory arteritides.

Neither presentation were suggestive of migraine-associated strokes. The negative antiphospholipid antibodies and antinuclear factor mitigated against the relevance of the antiphospholipid syndrome in this case. Likewise a procoagulopathy was excluded after the first admission.[2] The association of migraine and strokes raises the possible diagnosis of cerebral autosomal dominant arteriopathy with subcortical infarctions and leukoencephalopathy (CADASIL). An appropriate family history of migraine, strokes and dementia may not necessarily be obtained unless specifically sought. The diagnosis may be confirmed by the identification of mutations in the Notch3 gene on chromosome 19,[3] which encodes a calcium channel protein. However, the MRI brain scan in CADASIL reveals an extensive leukoencephalopathy which was absent in this patient.

Young onset stroke should also raise the possibility of an inborn error of metabolism. Whilst many of these may be characterized by clinical features outside the CNS, homocysteinuria[4] and mitochondrial disorders may manifest with stroke alone. Homocysteine levels in blood and urine are relatively easily detected. The mitochondrial encephalomyopathies can manifest with a wide spectrum of multisystem involvement.[5,6] One clini-cally defined subgroup, those with the MELAS (myopathy, encephalopa-thy lactic acidosis and stroke-like episodes), phenotype are known to present as young onset strokes, sometimes without any additional features of the syndrome. In this patient the history of migraine with aura and a maternal history of non-insulin dependent diabetes mellitus are suggestive of MELAS. The parieto-occipital area appears to be a site of predilection for MELAS associated strokes and their presence should always raise this as a possible diagnosis.

The patient had a left vastus lateralis muscle biopsy. This showed changes typical of a mitochondrial myopathy with ragged red, succinate dehydrogenase and cytochrome oxidase positive and negative fibers (Fig. 21.1). Subsequent molecular genetic analysis showed a point mutation (A3243G) in the mitochondrial DNA (mtDNA) transfer RNA for leucine (UUR) – the most common cause of MELAS.

MELAS is one of the primary mitochondrial disorders of oxidative phosphorylation and may be caused by a variety of different mtDNA mutations, including and number of different tRNA point mutations and deletions. However, the A3243G mutation accounts for the majority of cases. Affected patients may manifest in adolescence with short stature, limb myopathy, seizures and episodes of lactic acidosis. Additional features include non-insulin dependent diabetes mellitus and sensorineural deafness. The 'stroke-like' episodes may occur as part of the full

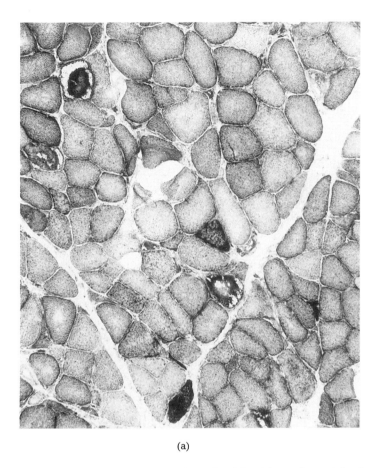

(a)

Fig. 21.1. Sequential sections of muscle stained for (a) succinate dehydrogenase (SDH) and (b) cytochrome oxidase (COX). The SDH stain shows several
fibers with increased accumulation of SDH activity representing the equivalent
of ragged red fibers. The COX stain shows that some of the SDH-positive fibers
also stain heavily for COX but some are also COX-negative. Characteristically
in MELAS cases the SDH-positive fibers are also COX-positive. However, in
other mitochondrial myopathies, e.g. CPEO and Kearns–Sayre, the SDH-positive fibers are COX-negative.

phenotype or, as with other features of MELAS, occur in isolation. The
clinical features of the strokes are, in general, indistinguishable from
embolic strokes although their pathogenesis is different. The 'strokes' in
MELAS do not conform to vascular territories. Pathological studies have
demonstrated abnormal mitochondria in intracerebral arterioles staining
strongly for SDH. Abnormal vascular tone and local biochemical derangements such as lactic acidosis and impaired ATP synthesis probably con-

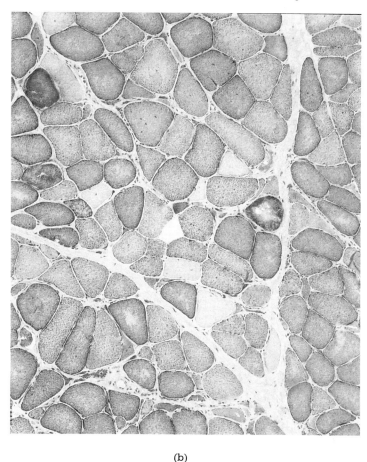

(b)

Fig. 21.1. (continued)

tribute together to neuronal dysfunction. The parieto-occipital lobes are preferentially affected and MRI scans show increased signal on T2-weighted images. A CT scan may demonstrate basal ganglia calcification in a proportion of MELAS patients.

Patients may have high lactate and lactate/pyruvate ratios in blood and/ or cerebrospinal fluid and this may be a useful clue to an underlying mitochondrial defect. Creatine kinase levels are often normal or only mildly elevated. Electromyography may show myopathic features but is often non-specific.

The point mutations causing MELAS may be detected in blood in a high proportion of patients, whilst the mtDNA mutation is invariably present in muscle. Thus a positive test for a mtDNA mutation in blood may be diagnostic, but a negative result does not exclude the diagnosis. If there is high clinical suspicion of an underlying mitochondrial myopathy, a muscle biopsy should be performed and molecular genetic studies undertaken on this tissue.

The diagnosis of mitochondrial disease in the context of stroke is important as this will influence future investigations and management. In the acute stage there is little to offer beyond the standard supportive care afforded to any stroke patient. Seizures and a lactic acidosis may accompany the stroke and should be treated as appropriate with anticonvulsants (avoiding sodium valproate because of its interaction with mitochondrial metabolism) and sodium bicarbonate. Persistent seizures and coma have been noted to improve in MELAS patients given steroids although the basis for this is unclear. Longer term, it is not known whether anti-platelet therapy provides MELAS patients any protection against further strokes. The use of ubiquinone (co-enzyme Q_{10}) may be of theoretical value in acting as a free radical scavenger and electron carrier, but there has been no formal clinical trial of such therapy.

Diagnosis

MELAS.

References

1. Silbert PL, Mokri B, Schievink WI. Headache and neck pain in spontaneous internal carotid and vertebral artery dissections. *Neurology* 1995; **45:** 1517–1522.
2. Zöller B, Dahlbäck B. Resistance to activated protein C caused by a Factor V gene mutation. *Curr Opin Hematol* 1995; **2:** 358–364.
3. Joutel A, Corpechot C, Ducros A, Vahedi K, Chabriat H, Mouton P et al. Notch 3 mutations in CADASIL, a hereditary adult-onset condition causing stroke and dementia. *Nature* 1996; **383:** 707–710.
4. Evers S, Koch HG, Grotemeyey KH, Lange B, Deufel T, Ringelstein EB. Features, symptoms and neurophysiological findings in stroke associated with hyperhomocysteinemia. *Arch Neurol* 1997; **54:** 1276–1282.
5. Leonard JV, Schapira AHV. Mitochondrial respiratory chain disorders I: mitochondrial DNA defects. *Lancet* 2000; **355:** 299–304.
6. Leonard JV, Schapira AHV. Mitochondrial respiratory chain disorders II: neurodegenerative disorders and nuclear gene defects. *Lancet* 2000; **355:** 389–394.

Weak legs with both neurogenic and myopathic features

At age 18, this man noted a postural tremor. He had been a University basketball player in high school. At age 26, in 1982, he was told his creatine kinase (CK) values were high in a routine checkup. He was otherwise asymptomatic until age 30, in 1986, when he had difficulty running. By 1993 he had difficulty climbing stairs. In 1999, he was using a cane and had difficulty rising from chairs. He had no weakness of arms or hands and noted muscle twitching only in his chin, arms and legs. The chin fasciculations increased after movement of the lips. He had no cramps and had not lost weight. There was no family history of consanguinity or similar disease. He had had three children; he and his wife carried the gene for alpha thalassemia.

In 1993, EMG showed signs of denervation in both legs. Serum CK activity was 4800, with increased serum values for other sarcoplasmic enzymes and myoglobin. In 1999, CK was 1487 (normal 40–285), CK-MB 18.6 (normal < 3.2) and AST-GOT was normal. Muscle biopsy showed large groups of atrophic fibers among normal-sized fibers and hypertrophic fibers. The atrophic fibers included both types 1 and 2. There was mild fiber-type grouping. Fibers with centrally located nuclei were moderately increased. A few target fibers, necrotic fibers, regenerating fibers and split fibers were seen. A few fibers contained rimmed vacuoles, most which were centrally located, suggesting that they were related to target formation. There was mild endomysial fibrosis and sparse lymphocytes infiltrated the endomysium. The features were primarily neurogenic with some myopathic features but no specific diagnostic changes and no metabolic accumulations (Fig. 22.1). Dystrophin stains gave a normal pattern.

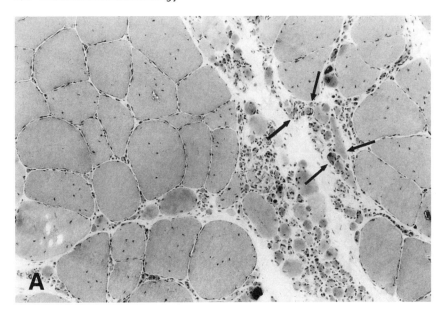

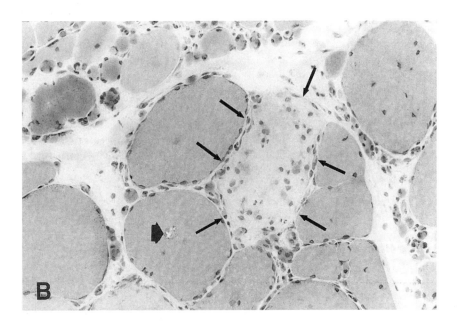

Fig. 22.1. Muscle biopsy. (A) The arrows outline one of several groups of atrophic fibers in this specimen, a pattern indicative of a neurogenic disorder. Many of the large fibers have centrally located nuclei, a feature that is typical of a chronic myopathy. (B) A necrotic muscle fiber has been invaded by macrophages (arrows), a 'myopathic' feature.

In 1999, findings on general examination were normal except for mild gynecomastia of which the patient was unaware. All cranial nerve functions were normal except that the mentalis was wasted and twitching. His speech was clear and the tongue was not atrophic or twitching. There were no snout or jaw reflexes. The postural tremor was prominent, but there was no weakness of wasting in arms or hands. His gait had a slightly waddling character and he had difficulty walking on heels or toes. There was weakness against resistance of proximal leg muscles but distal muscles were strong. Coarse fasciculation was seen in biceps, triceps and quadriceps. Tendon reflexes were normal in the arms, present with reinforcement at the knees and absent at the ankles. There were no Hoffmann or Babinski signs or clonus. Sensation was intact.

A diagnostic test was performed.

*   *   *

Discussion

This patient's illness raises the question of differentiating myopathic and neurogenic disease because of the high serum CK values and mixed myopathic–neurogenic pattern in the muscle biopsy. It also depends on the differential diagnosis of lower motor neuron diseases because of the widespread fasciculation and evidence of denervation in the EMG.

There are few diseases in which both muscle biopsy and EMG show both neurogenic and myopathic features. Among them are acid maltase deficiency, inclusion body myositis, facioscapulohumeral dystrophy, and scapuloperoneal muscular dystrophy. Diagnosis of acid maltase deficiency and inclusion body myositis depends on muscle biopsy findings that were lacking here. Facioscapulohumeral and scapuloperoneal muscular dystrophies are both characterized by the specific distribution of muscle weakness implied by the names; neither pattern of weakness was observed in this patient.

It therefore seems more fruitful to seek neurogenic diseases that may have myopathic features. High serum CK values are encountered in juvenile spinal muscular atrophy, the Kugelberg–Welander syndrome. They are also encountered in some patients with amyotrophic lateral sclerosis (ALS), including the purely lower motor neuron form called 'adult-onset progressive spinal muscular atrophy' (PSMA). However, high CK values do not identify a specific clinical form of ALS. Values as high as in the present case may also be seen in X-linked spinobulbar muscular atrophy (Kennedy syndrome, XSBMA). Presumably, high CK values could also be seen in an autoimmune peripheral neuropathy with myopathy, but there was no sensory loss here and nerve conduction velocities were normal. So, we are left with the three main forms of spinal muscular atrophy. Postural tremor occurs in children with spinal muscular atrophy (SMA) and probably also in later onset forms of SMA.

Muscle weakness here began at age 30, which is late for SMA but not impossible. Amyotrophic lateral sclerosis, even the PSMA form, starts before age 40 in only 10% of cases and there was no suggestion of an upper motor neuron disorder. Amyotrophic lateral sclerosis therefore seems unlikely. Another possibility is the Kennedy syndrome, which is X-linked, recessive. There were no other known affected family members, but none had been examined. The two diagnostic clues here may be the gynecomastia and the twitching in the mentalis, increasing after lip movements. Both point heavily to XSBMA and nothing in the record is inconsistent with that diagnosis.

Cases had been described earlier, but the full description, including X-linkage, was given in 1968 by Kennedy et al.[1] Although the clinical abnormalities are restricted to the motor system, Harding et al.[2] found that sural nerve potentials may be absent and others[3,4] have also found abnormalities of sensory conduction. However, sensory symptoms are exceptional and, at autopsy, Sobue and colleagues[5,6] found the brunt of the pathology in motor neurons with sparing of the sensory neurons and sparse pathology in the sural nerve. There seemed to be a distal sensory axonopathy. In contrast to ALS, loss of motor neurons was not accompanied by gliosis.

Studies of central conduction exonerated the upper motor neuron but confirmed the asymptomatic involvement of sensory neurons.[7] Similarly, there was no evidence of upper motor neuron disorder in peristimulus time histograms after magnetic stimulation of the cortex,[8] or in magnetic resonance spectroscopy[9] and specific post-mortem study showed no loss of myelinated fiber density in the corticospinal tracts.[10]

Warner et al.[11] tabulated the clinical manifestations in 75 affected members of 31 reported families (Table 22.1). Among the findings in more than 90% of affected individuals were facial weakness, proximal more than distal limb weakness, perioral fasciculation, and visible limb fasciculations. Findings in 80–89% included loss of knee and ankle jerks and lingual fasciculation. Findings in 70–79% were cramps, dysarthria, and paternity. Vibration was the only sensory modality affected and that was recorded in 14%. Gynecomastia was not consistently noted, but seemed to be present in about half the cases. Hausmanowa-Petrusewicz et al.[12] noted the frequency of postural tremor as they had in children with SMA, and others have mentioned a high frequency of postural tremor. The origin of the tremor is not clear. Longevity seems little affected and mechanical ventilation is barely mentioned, but some patients lose the ability to walk.

Perhaps the two most important diagnostic findings in the present case were the gynecomastia (which is common in the general population but more common in Kennedy disease) and the perioral fasciculation. Olney et al.[13] describe repetitive grouped discharges after mild activation

Table 22.1. Manifestations of Kennedy–Alter–Sung disease: 79 affected members of 31 families. From Warner et al.[11]

Symptom or sign	No. abnormal/no. studied	%
Cramps	43/61	70
Dysarthria	62/79	78
Face weak	60/63	95
Proximal > distal limb weakness	76/79	96
Knee jerks, ankle jerks absent	57/67	85
Tongue fasciculation	65/78	83
Perioral fasciculation	60/66	91
Limb fasciculation	76/78	97
Impaired vibration sensation	9/63	14
Paternity	49/68	72
Gynecomastia	39*	

* Number studied not stated.

of the facial muscles and some investigators consider these movements almost pathognomonic of Kennedy disease.[14] These signs are common in SBMA but so rare in ALS that the diagnosis of Kennedy syndrome seems almost forced upon us.

The diagnostic test

The mean number of CAG repeats in normal people is in the range 11–38. Analysis of the patient's DNA gave a value of 49 and is diagnostic of X-linked spinobulbar muscular atrophy (XSBMA) or Kennedy disease. The lack of other affected family members could be explained by any of three possibilities: (1) The patient's mother is the carrier of a new mutation. (2) The patient's germ line has had a new mutation. (3) Other members of the family are affected in an X-linked pattern but their conditions are mild and they have not been examined.

Further discussion

Kennedy disease was the first to be identified as one of triplet repeats, an observation made by Fischbeck and his colleagues in 1991.[15] At least 14 other diseases are now in that category, including spinocerebellar ataxias, Huntington disease, myotonic dystrophy, Friedreich ataxia and oculopharyngeal muscular dystrophy. These clinically and pathologically diverse diseases have one feature in common: the longer the repeat, the earlier the age at onset. The repeats are also 'unstable,' which means they can expand or contract in different individuals. Expansion is more common so that the age at onset tends to be earlier in successive generations, a phenomenon called anticipation. The longer the number of repeats the more severe the clinical syndrome, so that 'potentiation' is also seen in succeeding generations. However, there is no absolute relation between the size of the expansion and the severity of symptoms, which may vary even in siblings with expansions of similar size.[16]

Fischbeck et al.[17] have summarized the molecular genetics. The gene is located at Xq11-12. The expanded repeat is located in the first exon of the androgen receptor gene, but loss of androgen receptor function does not seem to be the main problem. Dysfunctional mutations in this gene result in testicular feminization or androgen insensitivity without any motor neuron disorder. Instead, XSBMA is attributed to a toxic gain of function that is induced by the polyglutamine expansion encoded in the triplet repeat. Transgenic mice have been produced and, like other triplet repeat diseases, the presence of a truncated protein (rather than the entire protein) has a pronounced effect in inducing the phenotype. The truncated protein may be responsible for the toxicity of the mutation.[18] Like other trinucleotide repeat diseases, XSBMA is characterized histologically by the presence of nuclear inclusions made up of the polyglutamine-containing protein. The neuronal inclusions are ubiquitinated. They have been found in humans, transgenic mice, and transfected cells in culture. Gene products with expansions of the triplet repeat are substrates for cleavage by caspases, the 'cysteine protease cell death executioners.'[19] Despite this progress, there is still no effective treatment. Testosterone may increase scores in tests of muscle strength[20] but does not improve quality of life and the effect may be a nonspecific androgenic effect on muscle, normal or abnormal.

Discovery of the molecular fault has had a clinical impact. First, it resolves diagnostic problems, as in the present case. Second, testing populations of ALS patients indicates that about 2% of them actually have XSBMA.[21] Third, DNA analysis has indicated that clinically similar syndromes may lack the CAG expansion; one such family showed autosomal dominant inheritance.[22]

Diagnosis

X-linked spinobulbar muscular atrophy.

References

1. Kennedy WR, Alter M, Sung JH. Progressive proximal spinal and bulbar muscular atrophy of late onset: a sex-linked trait. *Neurology* 1968; **18:** 671–680.
2. Harding AE, Thomas PK, Baraister M, Bradbury PG, Morgan-Hughes JA, Posford JR. X-linked recessive bulbospinal neuronopathy: a report of 10 cases. *J Neurol Neurosurg Psychiatry* 1982; **45:** 1012–1019.

3. Ferrante MA, Wilbourn AJ. The characteristic electrodiagnostic features of Kennedy's disease. *Muscle Nerve* 1997; **20**: 323–329.
4. Antonini G, Gragnani F, Romaniello A et al. Sensory involvement in spinal–bulbar muscular atrophy (Kennedy's disease). *Muscle Nerve* 2000; **23**: 252–258.
5. Sobue G, Hashizume Y, Mukai E et al. X-linked recessive bulbospinal neuronopathy. *Brain* 1989; **112**: 209–232.
6. Li M, Sobue G, Doyu M et al. Primary sensory neurons in X-linked recessive bulbospinal neuronopathy: histopathology and androgen gene expression. *Muscle Nerve* 1995; **18**: 301–308.
7. Kachi T, Sobue G, Sobue J. Central motor and sensory conduction in X-linked recessive bulbospinal neuronopathy. *J Neurol Neurosurg Psychiatry* 1992; **55**: 394–397.
8. Weber M, Eisen A. Assessment of upper and lower motor neurons in Kennedy's disease. Implications for corticomotorneuronal PSTH studies. *Muscle Nerve* 1999; **22**: 299–306.
9. Kaaitzky J, Block W, Mellies JK. Proton magnetic resonance spectroscopy in Kennedy syndrome. *Arch Neurol* 1999; **56**: 1465–1471.
10. Terao S, Sobue G, Li M et al. The lateral corticospinal tract and spinal ventral horn in X-linked recessive spinal and bulbar muscular atrophy: a quantitative study. *Acta Neuropathol* 1997; **93**: 1–6.
11. Warner CL, Servidei S, Lange DJ, Miller E, Lovelace RE, Rowland LP. X-linked spinal muscular atrophy (Kennedy's syndrome): a kindred with hypobetalipoproteinemia. *Arch Neurol* 1990, **47**: 1117–1120.
12. Hausmanowa-Petrusewicz I, Borkowska J, Janczewski Z. X-linked adult form of spinal muscular atrophy. *J Neurol* 1983; **229**: 175–178.
13. Olney RK, Aminoff MJ, So YT. Clinical and electrodiagnostic features of X-linked recessive bulbospinal neuronopathy. *Neurology* 1991; **41**: 823–828.
14. Meriggoli MN, Rowin J, Sanders DB. Distinguishing clinical and electrodiagnostic features of X-lined bulbospinal neuronopathy. *Muscle Nerve* 1999; **22**: 1693–1697.
15. La Spada AR, Wilson EM, Lubahn DB, Harding AE, Fischbeck KE. Androgen receptor gene mutations in X-linked spinal and bulbar muscular atrophy. *Nature* 1991; **352**: 77–79.
16. Shimada N, Sobue G, Doyu M et al. X-linked recessive bulbospinal neuronopathy: clinical phenotypes and CAG repeat size in androgen receptor gene. *Muscle Nerve* 1995; **18**: 1378–1384.
17. Fischbeck KH, Lieberman A, Bailey CK, Abel A, Merry DE. Androgen receptor mutation in Kennedy's disease. *Phil Trans R Soc Lond B* 1999; **354**: 1075–1078.
18. Butler R, Leigh PN, McPhaul MJ, Gallo J-M. Truncated forms of the androgen receptor are associated with polyglutamine expansion in X-linked spinal and bulbar muscular atrophy. *Hum Mol Genet* 1998; **7**: 121–127.
19. Ellerby LM, Hackam AS, Propp SS et al. Kennedy's disease: caspase cleavage of the androgen receptor is a crucial event in cytotoxicity. *J Neurochem* 1999; **72**: 185–192.
20. Goldenberg JN, Bradley WG. Testosterone therapy and the pathogenesis of Kennedy's disease (X-linked bulbospinal muscular atrophy). *J Neurol Sci* 1996; **135**: 158–161.

21. Paraboosingh JS, Figlewicz DA, Krizus A et al. Spinobulbar muscular atrophy can mimic ALS; the importance of genetic testing in male patients with atypical ALS. *Neurology* 1997; **49:** 568–572.
22. Ikezoe K, Yosimura T, Taniwaki T et al. Autosomal dominant familial spinal and bulbar muscular atrophy with gynecomastia. *Neurology* 1999; **53:** 2187–2189.

Worsening tension headache

Clinical history and examination

A 30-year-old man in good previous health presented with an 8-day history of worsening severe headache. He had no prior history of migraine, but he did have occasional episodic tension-type headaches. The current headache began like his typical tension-type headache, but became progressively worse. He went to the emergency department at the local hospital. His vital signs, including his temperature, and his general neurologic examination were within normal limits. No sinus tenderness was present. A diagnosis of tension-type headache was made and he was prescribed acetaminophen with codeine. His pain was unrelieved by the prescribed analgesic and he returned to the emergency room. A white count of 14 000 was noted and a computed tomography (CT) was performed and interpreted as within normal limits, and he was again discharged.

When seen again, the patient was complaining of an incapacitating, pressing, and at times throbbing headache, located across his forehead and the top of his head. It was not associated with nausea, vomiting, blurry vision, or double vision, but was aggravated by movement. He did not have back pain or a stiff neck. He had photophobia, but no phonophobia or tinnitus.

He was alert, oriented, lucid, and in obvious distress. His blood pressure was 122/80, pulse 76, and temperature 98.6°F. Straight leg raising test was negative and his neck was supple. Examination was normal. Investigations were undertaken.

Lumbar puncture revealed an opening pressure of 230 mm of cerebrospinal fluid with 140 RBCs/mm^3 (the tap was slightly traumatic) and 20 WBCs/mm^3 (37% segs, 40% lymphs, 23% monos). Cryptococcal antigen, gram stain, and bacterial and fungal cultures were negative.

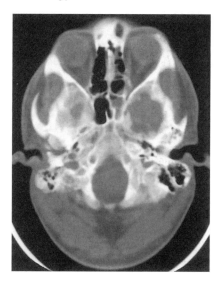

Fig. 23.1. Computed tomography scan showing opacification of left sphenoid sinus and left ethmoid sinus.

Protein was 113 mg/dl, glucose 61 mg/dl, and IgG 7.1 mg/dl. Angiotensin-converting enzyme was 10 U/l (normal 8–52 U/l). WBC was 11 300 with 86.5% granulocytes.

Retrospective review of the outpatient CT scan that was reported as normal showed opacification of the left sphenoid sinus and involvement of the left ethmoid sinus (Fig. 23.1). Magnetic resonance imaging (MRI) showed progression to complete opacification of the left sphenoid sinus and partial opacification of the right sphenoid sinus. Moderate left ethmoid and minimal left frontal sinus involvement was noted (Fig. 23.2a). Magnetic resonance imaging with gadolinium showed diffuse pathologic contrast enhancement over the paranasal sinus and along the floor of the anterior and left middle cranial fossa (Fig. 23.2b).

*   *   *

Discussion

The patient was admitted and treated with cefotaxime sodium 2 g intravenously every 8 hours for 10 days. The headache was markedly improved after 2 days, and was gone after 4 days. He was discharged on cefuroxime 500 mg t.i.d. and metronidazole 500 mg t.i.d. for 2 weeks. At follow-up examination 2 weeks after discharge, he was well, with no recurrence of the throbbing headache and only an occasional tension-type headache.

Sinusitis affects an estimated 35 million people. The prevalence of acute sinusitis appears to be increasing, according to data from the National

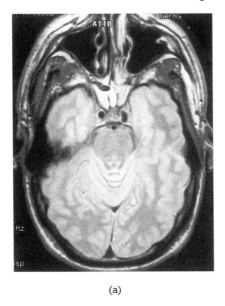

(a)

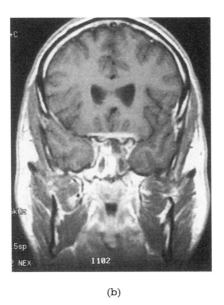

(b)

Fig. 23.2. (a) Magnetic resonance imaging scan showing complete opacification of the left sphenoid sinus and partial opacification of the right sphenoid sinus. Moderate involvement of the left ethmoid and minimal involvement of the left frontal sinus was also seen. (b) Gadolinium-enhanced MRI showing pathological enhancement over the paranasal sinus and along the floor of the anterior and left middle cranial fossa.

Ambulatory Medical Care Survey, from 0.2% of diagnoses at office visits in 1990 to 0.4% of diagnoses at office visits in 1995.[1]

The primary functions of the nasal passages are humidification, warming, and removal of particulate material from the inspired air. The paranasal sinuses are airfilled cavities that communicate with the nasal airway. They are lined with pseudostratified ciliated epithelium, which is covered by a thin layer of mucus that receives the largest deposits of inhaled large particulate matter. The cilia and this mucous layer are in constant motion in a predetermined direction. Mucus and debris are transported towards the ostia by the beating of the cilia and are expelled into the nasal airway.[2–4] Ciliary dysfunction or ostial obstruction is necessary for bacterial proliferation and the development of sinus infection. Systemic diseases that predispose to sinusitis include cystic fibrosis (with impaired mucus production), immune deficiency, bronchiectasis, and the immobile cilia syndrome (with impaired mucus transport).

All sinuses normally contain anaerobic bacteria and more than one-third harbor both anaerobic and aerobic organisms. Bacterial infection of the sinuses is generally effectively cleared by this mechanism. If the sinus ostia are obstructed, mucociliary flow is interrupted. Obstruction causes the oxygen tension within the sinus to decrease and the carbon dioxide tension to increase. This anaerobic environment can facilitate bacterial growth.[4]

The sinuses are involved in nearly 90% of viral upper respiratory infections. In patients with a common cold and no previous history of rhinosinusitis, 87% had maxillary sinus abnormalities, 65% ethmoid sinus abnormalities, and 30–40% frontal or sphenoid sinus abnormalities on CT. The abnormalities are most likely due to highly viscid secretions in the sinuses.

Wolff showed that the sinuses themselves are relatively insensitive to pain.[5] McAuliffe and associates,[6] using touch, pressure, and electrical stimulation, found that the nasal turbinates and sinus ostia were much more sensitive than the mucosal lining of the septum and the paranasal sinuses. Most of the pain that was elicited was referred pain.

The physical examination may not be helpful in the diagnosis of sinusitis. Not all patients are febrile and sinus tenderness is not always present. Pus is not always seen in sphenoid sinusitis. Transillumination of the sinuses has low sensitivity and specificity[7] and routine anterior rhinoscopy performed with a headlight and nasal speculum allows only limited inspection of the anterior nasal cavity.

Computed tomography or MRI is necessary to definitively diagnose sphenoid sinusitis because plain X-rays are nondiagnostic in about 26% of cases.[8] The mucosa of the sinus approximates the bone so closely that it cannot be visualized on CT. Therefore, any soft tissue bulge in the sinus is abnormal.[9] Computed tomography is still the gold standard for the diagnosis of sphenoid sinus disease; MRI is an adjunct. A major problem is the failure to look at and comment on the sinuses in patients referred for head CT, as seen in our case. Physicians should specifically request imaging of the sphenoid sinus.

Diagnostic endoscopy with the flexible fiberoptic rhinoscopy allows direct visualization of the nasal passages and sinus drainage areas (ostiomeatal complex) and is complementary to CT or MRI. Infection is easily diagnosed if purulent material is seen emanating from the sinus drainage region. Mucosal sinus thickening is frequently present in normal, non-symptomatic patients. In these cases, endoscopy should be positive before a diagnosis of sinusitis can be made.[4,10] Sphenoid sinusitis is an exception to this generalization.

Endoscopy should be considered when a sinus related problem is suspected in a patient who fails to respond to conservative medical treatment and whose CT or MRI is inconclusive. Some use endoscopy prior to neuroimaging. The combination of negative neuroimaging and endoscopy usually, but not always, rules out sinus disease.[3]

In 1996, the American Academy of Otolaryngology – Head and Neck Surgery standardized the terminology for paranasal infections.[11] The term rhinosinusitis was felt to be more appropriate than sinusitis since rhinitis typically precedes sinusitis, purulent sinusitis without rhinitis is rare, the mucosa of the nose and sinuses are contiguous, and symptoms of nasal obstruction and discharge are prominent in sinusitis.[12] Rhinosinusitis is divided into four categories based on the temporal course and the signs and symptoms of the disease (Table 23.1): acute rhinosinusitis, subacute rhinosinusitis, recurrent acute rhinosinusitis, and chronic rhinosinusitis.[13]

Nasal congestion, purulent nasal discharge, and facial tenderness and pain are common manifestations of acute sinus infections. Other 'classic' signs and symptoms include anosmia, pain upon mastication, and halitosis. While fever is present in about 50% of adults and 60% of children and headache is common, the symptoms of headache, facial pain, and fever are often of minimal value in the diagnosis of sinusitis. Williams et al.[14] looked at the sensitivity and specificity of individual symptoms in making the diagnosis of sinusitis. No single item was both sensitive and specific. Maxillary toothache was highly specific (93%), but only 11% of the patients had this symptom. Logistic regression analysis showed five independent predictors of sinusitis: maxillary toothache (odds ratio 2.9), abnormal transillumination (odds ratio 2.7, sensitivity 73%, specificity 54%), poor response to decongestants (odds ratio 2.4), purulent discharge (odds ratio 2.9), and colored nasal discharge (odds ratio 2.2). The low specificity is due to lack of descriptive features of the headache.

One proposed classification system is based on major and minor clinical criteria. The major symptoms are purulent anterior or posterior nasal discharge, nasal congestion, facial pain or pressure, and fever. Minor symptoms are cough, headache (not otherwise specified), halitosis, and earache.[15] A diagnosis using these criteria requires two major criteria or one major and two minor criteria. However, none of these criteria are both

Table 23.1. Classification of adult rhinosinusitis.

Classification	Duration	Strong history	Include in differential	Special notes
Acute	≤4 weeks	≥ 2 major factors, one major factor and two minor factors, or nasal purulence on examination	One major factor or ≥ 2 minor factors	Fever or facial pain does not constitute a suggestive history in the absence of other nasal signs or symptoms; consider acute bacterial rhinosinusitis if symptoms worsen after five days, persist for > 10 days, or are out of proportion to those typically associated with viral infection
Subacute	4–12 weeks	Same as chronic	Same as chronic	Complete resolution after effective medical therapy
Recurrent acute	≥ 4 episodes per year, with each episode lasting ≥7–10 days and no intervening signs and symptoms of chronic rhinosinusitis	Same as acute		
Chronic	≥ 12 weeks	≥ 2 major factors, one major factor and two minor factors, or nasal purulence on examination	One major factor or ≥ 2 minor factors	Facial pain does not constitute a suggestive history in the absence of other nasal signs or symptoms
Acute exacerbations of chronic	Sudden worsening of chronic rhinosinusitis, with return to baseline after treatment			

sensitive and specific enough for diagnosis. It has been suggested that highly specific symptoms such as facial erythema, maxillary toothache, or symptoms that persist for more than 10 days warrant a diagnosis and treatment.[16] The Agency for Healthcare Policy and Research evidence report,[1] based on limited evidence, suggested that clinical criteria (i.e. three or four of the following symptoms: purulent rhinorrhea with unilateral predominance, local pain with unilateral predominance, bilateral purulent rhinorrhea, and pus in the nasal cavity) may have a diagnostic accuracy similar to that of sinus radiography (Table 23.2).

Sphenoid sinusitis is an uncommon infection that accounts for approximately 3% of all cases of acute sinusitis. It is usually accompanied by pansinusitis. In contrast to other paranasal sinus infections, sphenoid sinusitis is frequently misdiagnosed, since the sphenoid sinus is not accessible to direct clinical examination even with the flexible endoscope and is not adequately visualized with routine sinus X-rays.[8] While sphenoid sinusitis is an uncommon cause of headache, it is potentially associated with significant morbidity and mortality and requires early identification and aggressive management.[8,17,18]

Headache is the most common symptom of acute sphenoid sinusitis; it is present in all patients who are able to complain about it. Standing, walking, bending, or coughing aggravates it; it often interferes with sleep and is poorly relieved by narcotics. Its location is variable. Vertex headache is rare; frontal, occipital, or temporal headache or a combination of these locations is most common. Periorbital pain is common. This is in contrast to the common teaching that retro-orbital or vertex headache is the most common presenting symptom of sphenoid sinusitis.[8,17–21]

Nausea and vomiting frequently occur during an attack of acute ethmoid sinusitis, but nasal discharge, stuffiness, and postnasal drip are unusual. Fever occurs in over one-half of patients with acute sphenoid sinusitis. Isolated sphenoid sinusitis has been subclassified into four groups (inflammatory, neoplastic, fibro-osseous disorders, and miscellaneous) in a series of 132 cases.[22] Headache, visual loss, and cranial nerve palsy prevalence was determined in each group. Headache occurred in 98% of the inflammatory lesions, 90% of the benign tumors, and 71% of the malignant tumors. Visual disturbances (blurred vision and loss of visual acuity) were found in 12% of inflammatory lesions, 60% of benign tumors, and 50% of malignant neoplasms. Sixth cranial nerve palsy occurred in 6% of the inflammatory and 50% of the neoplastic cases. Eyelid ptosis (due to third-nerve involvement) occurred in 7.5% of the cases. Other symptoms included cerebrospinal fluid leaks, epistaxis, meningitis, and proptosis. Four patients with fibro-osseous disorder presented with headache.

Sphenoid sinusitis should be included in the differential diagnosis of acute or subacute headache. It may be mistaken for frontal or ethmoid sinusitis, aseptic meningitis, brain abscess, or septic thrombophlebitis. It can mimic trigeminal neuralgia, migraine, carotid artery aneurysm, or brain tumor.[8,17,18] Other causes of sphenoid sinus disease include mucoceles and benign or malignant tumors.[22]

The clinical features of a severe, intractable, new onset headache that interferes with sleep, increases in severity, has no specific location, and is not relieved by simple analgesics should alert one to the diagnosis of sphenoid sinusitis. Pain or paresthesias in the facial distribution of the

Table 23.2. Acute sinus headache – diagnostic criteria.

A. Purulent discharge in the nasal passage either spontaneous or by suction
B. Pathologic findings in one or more of the following tests:
   1. X-ray examination
   2. Computed tomography or magnetic resonance imaging
   3. Transillumination
C. Simultaneous onset of headache and sinusitis
D. Headache location:
   1. In acute frontal sinusitis headache is located directly over the sinus and may radiate to the vertex or behind the eyes
   2. In acute maxillary sinusitis headache is located over the antral area and may radiate to the upper teeth or the forehead
   3. In acute ethmoiditis headache is located between the eyes and may radiate to the temporal area
   4. In acute sphenoiditis headache is located in the occipital area, the vertex, the frontal region, or behind the eyes
E. Headache disappears after treatment of acute sinusitis

fifth nerve and photophobia or eye tearing are suggestive of sphenoid sinusitus.[8,17,18,20,21,23]

Sinus infection can result in acute suppurative meningitis, subdural or epidural abscess, and brain abscess. In addition, osteomyelitis and subperiosteal abscess can occur. Infection of the ethmoid and, to a lesser extent, the sphenoid sinuses is responsible for orbital complications, which include edema, orbital cellulitis, and subperiosteal and orbital abscess. Sinusitis thus can be a life-threatening condition and if neglected or mismanaged can lead to intracranial complications.[24] In a review of patients admitted to the University of Virginia Health Sciences Center with a diagnosis of intracranial suppuration between 1992 and 1997, 15 patients were found who had 22 suppurative intracranial complications of sinusitis. These included epidural abscess (23%), subdural empyema (18%), meningitis (18%), cerebral abscess (14%), superior sagittal sinus thrombosis (9%), cavernous sinus thrombosis (9%), and osteomyelitis (9%). The diagnosis of suppurative intracranial complications of sinusitis requires a high index of suspicion and confirmation by imaging.

Sphenoid sinusitis is associated with most major central nervous system complications, which include bacterial meningitis, cavernous sinus thrombosis, subdural abscess, cortical vein thrombosis, ophthalmoplegia, and pituitary insufficiency.[8,17,18,25,26] In addition, sphenoid sinusitis can present as an aseptic meningitis due to the presence of a parameningeal focus.[26] Patients can present with the complications of sphenoid sinusitis, including visual loss mimicking optic neuritis, multiple cranial nerve palsies, or papilledema. Sudden onset as a result of cavernous sinus thrombosis can mimic the thunderclap headache that is usually associated with a subarachnoid hemorrhage.[27]

Øktedalen and Lilleas reported on four patients with ethmoid sinusitis who were admitted to an infectious disease department with meningitis, sepsis, and orbital cellulitis.[28] In the Lew et al.[17] series, six of 16 acute cases had meningitis, five had cavernous sinus thrombosis, one had cortical vein thrombosis, one had unilateral ophthalmoplegia, and one had orbital cellulitis.[17] Eight of Kibblewhite's 14 patients had complications on admission.[18] None of the Goldman et al.[8] patients had complications. The difference in the complication rate is a result of selection bias: the patients studied by Goldman et al.[8] were retrieved from emergency room records and those studied by Lew et al.,[17] Øktedalen and Lilleas,[28] and Kibblewhite et al.[18] from inpatient records.[8,18,28]

Management goals for the treatment of sinusitis include: (1) treatment of bacterial infection; (2) reduction of ostial swelling; (3) sinus drainage; and (4) maintenance of sinus ostial patency.

Sphenoid sinusitis without complications may be managed with high-dose intravenous antibiotics and topical and systemic decongestants for 24 hours.[8,18] If the fever (if present) and the headache do not start to improve or if any complications are present or develop, sphenoid sinus drainage is indicated.[29] Gilain et al.[30] reviewed 12 cases of isolated sphenoid sinus disease secondary to chronic inflammatory sinusitis (seven cases), mucoceles (two cases), aspergillus lesions (two cases), and an isolated polyp (one case). All the patients in this series were treated with functional endoscopic sphenoidotomy and improved. They were also treated with appropriate postoperative antibiotics, nasal irrigation, oral corticosteroids, and washing and cleaning of the nasal cavity weekly for 4 weeks.

Diagnosis

Sinusitis.

References

1. Agency for Healthcare Policy and Research. Diagnosis and treatment of acute bacterial rhinosinusitis. Summary. Evidence Report/Technology Assessment No. 9, 1999.
2. Reilly JS. The sinusitis cycle. *Otolaryngol Head Neck Surg* 1990; **103**: 856–862.
3. Zinreich SJ. Paranasal sinus imaging. *Otolaryngol Head Neck Surg* 1990; **103**: 863–869.
4. McCaffrey TV. Functional endoscopic sinus surgery: an overview. *Mayo Clin Proc* 1993; **68**: 675–677.
5. Wolff HG. *Wolff's Headache and other Head Pain*. Oxford: Oxford University Press, 1948.
6. McAuliffe GW, Goodell H, Wolff HG. Experimental studies on headache: pain from the nasal and paranasal structures. *Res Publ Assoc Res Nerv Ment Dis* 1943; **23**: 185–206.
7. Stafford CT. The clinician's view of sinusitis. *Otolaryngol Head Neck Surg* 1990; **103**: 870–875.

8. Goldman GE, Fontanarosa PB, Anderson JM. Isolated sphenoid sinusitis. *Am J Emerg Med* 1993; **11**: 235–238.

9. Schatz CJ, Becker TS. Normal CT anatomy of the paranasal sinuses. *Radiol Clin North Am* 1984; **22**: 107–118.

10. Kennedy DW. Surgical update. *Otolaryngol Head Neck Surg* 1990; **103**: 884–886.

11. Benninger MS, Anon J, Mabry RL. The medical management of rhinosinusitis (Review). Report of the Rhinosinusitis Task Force Committee Meeting. *Otolaryngol Head Neck Surg* 1997; **117**: S41–S49.

12. Slavin RG. Nasal polyps and sinusitis. *JAMA* 1997; 278: 1849–1854.

13. Lanza DC, Kennedy DW. Adult rhinosinusitis defined. *Otolaryngol Head Neck Surg* 1997; **117**: S1–S7.

14. Williams JW, Simel DL, Roberts L et al. Clinical evaluation of sinusitis. *Ann Intern Med* 1992; **117**: 705–710.

15. Shapiro GG, Rachelefsky GS. Introduction and definition of sinusitis. *J Allergy Clin Immunol* 1992; **90**: 417–418.

16. International Rhinosinusitis Advisory Board. Infectious rhinosinusitis in adults: classification, etiology, and management. *Ear Nose Throat J* 1997; **76**: S5–S22.

17. Lew D, Southwick FS, Montgomery WW et al. Sphenoid sinusitis: a review of 30 cases. *N Engl J Med* 1983; **19**: 1149–1154.

18. Kibblewhite DJ, Cleland J, Mintz DR. Acute sphenoid sinusitis: management strategies. *J Otolaryngol* 1988; **17**: 159–163.

19. Urquhart AC, Fung G, McIntosh WA. Isolated sphenoiditis: a diagnostic problem. *J Laryngol Otol* 1989; **103**: 526–527.

20. Nordeman L, Lucid E. Sphenoid sinusitis, a cause of debilitating headache. *J Emerg Med*, 1990; **8**: 557–559.

21. Deans JAJ, Welch AR. Acute isolated sphenoid sinusitis: a disease with complications. *J Laryngol Otol* 1991; **105**: 1072–1074.

22. Lawson W, Reino AJ. Isolated sphenoid sinus disease: an analysis of 132 cases. *Laryngoscope* 1997; **107**: 1590–1595.

23. Turkewitz D, Keller R. Acute headache in childhood: a case of sphenoid sinusitis. *Pediatr Emerg Care* 1987; **3**: 155–157.

24. Singh B, VanDellen J, Ramjettan S et al. Sinogenic intracranial complications. *J Laryngol Otol* 1995; **109**: 945–950.

25. Sofferman RA. Cavernous sinus thrombophlebitis secondary to sphenoid sinusitis. *Laryngoscope* 1983; **93**: 797–800.

26. Brook I, Overturf GD, Steinberg EA, Hawkins DB. Acute sphenoid sinusitis presenting as aseptic meningitis: a pachymeningitis syndrome. *Int J Pediatr Otorhinolaryngol* 1982; **4**: 77–81.

27. Dale BAB, Mackenzie IJ. The complications of sphenoid sinusitis. *J Laryngol Otol* 1983; **97**: 661–670.

28. Øktedalen O, Lilleas F. Septic complications to sphenoidal sinus infection. *Scand J Infect Dis* 1992; **24**: 353–356.

29. Druce HM. Adjuncts to medical management of sinusitis. *Otolaryngol Head Neck Surg* 1990; **103**: 880–883.

30. Gilain L, Aidan D, Coste A et al. Functional endoscopic sinus surgery for isolated sphenoid sinus disease. *Head Neck*, 1994; **16**: 433–437.

Acute vertigo and ataxia

Clinical history and examination

A 54-year-old left-handed man was admitted because of acute vertigo and ataxia. He admitted alcohol abuse. Three days prior to admission, he experienced sudden onset of vertigo, inability to stand, and poor balance; he crawled to the bathroom and vomited several times. The next day he noted dysarthria and diplopia on looking to the left. He was clumsy and could not write or feed himself. The vertigo was exacerbated by any movement of the head. The symptoms worsened progressively. He denied numbness, tingling, hearing loss, tinnitus, or dysphagia. The last drink he had was 1–2 days prior to the onset of symptoms. He unintentionally lost 20 lbs in the preceding 6 months.

Past medical history included the removal of small hard masses from each breast at age 40. The biopsy results were not available. He had a gun shot wound to the chest and stab wound to the neck at age 25. He had one sister with dysarthria and ataxia that were attributed to a 'stroke' at about age 50. He drinks regularly about 12 bottles of beer a day, and he was a 40-pack/year cigarette smoker. He denied drug use. He took a histamine H2-receptor inhibitor for occasional epigastric discomfort. He had not traveled outside Texas and Louisiana, and had no history of tick bites.

The pulse rate was 80, respiratory rate 16, blood pressure 180/100 mmHg, and temperature, 36.7°C. General examination showed a 5 mm submental node, a well-healed surgical scar on the left breast, and purulent discharge was noted from a scar above the right nipple. The lungs, heart, abdomen, external genitalia, rectum and extremities were unremarkable.

Neurological examination revealed normal mental and language functions. He had a left sixth nerve palsy and bilateral fast rotatory nystagmus, more pronounced on left lateral gaze. He was dysarthric. Bilateral marked dysmetria was most noted with finger–nose–finger and heel–shin testing; fine motor movements and rapid alternating movements

Table 24.1. The patient developed transient lymphocytic pleocytosis of the CSF.

Date	RBC (per mm^3)	WBC (per mm^3)	Lymphocytes	Total protein (mg/dl)	Glucose (mg/dl)
12 April 1999	7–5	279–321	90–91	47	70
20 April 1999	97–24	245–126	81–86	55	60
14 July 1999	5–2	6–7	96–98	39	58

were impaired bilaterally. He was ataxic, unable to stand or walk without support. Otherwise muscle strength, tone, tendon reflexes, and sensation were unremarkable.

The following were normal or negative: complete blood cell counts, serum electrolytes, liver function tests, folate, B12, thyroid-stimulating hormone, erythrocyte sedimentation rate, angiotensin-converting enzyme, and urine analysis, serum RPR and MHA-TP for syphilis, blood alcohol level and ELISA for human immunodeficiency virus. Urine toxicology screening was positive for marijuana. Chest radiography showed small left base atelectasis, bullet fragments, and old rib fracture. Examination of the cerebrospinal fluid (CSF) revealed a predominantly lymphocytic pleocytosis (Table 24.1). Cerebrospinal fluid VDRL, toxoplasma and cyto-megalovirus titers, cryptococcus antigen were nonreactive; gram stain and culture, fungal culture and acid-fast bacilli smear were negative. The IgG synthetic rate and index were consistent with intrathecal synthesis of IgG; oligoclonal bands were present. Cytological examinations of CSF performed twice were negative for malignant cells and showed reactive lymphocytes. Computed tomography and MRI of the brain with and without contrast material showed diffuse atrophy (Fig. 24.1).

Transesophageal echocardiogram and carotid Doppler studies were normal. Magnetic resonance angiography and percutaneous four-vessel cerebral angiography revealed no evidence of vasculitis but there was mild right internal carotid artery stenosis at the bulb. Computed tomography of the abdomen and pelvis was normal. Computed tomography of the chest showed a 9 mm nodule in the left upper lobe, bilateral basal atelectasis, evidence of emphysema and several small (less than 1 cm) lymph nodes of no clinical significance. Mammogram was normal. Biopsy from the right breast scar demonstrated acute and chronic inflammation. Prostate-specific antigen, carcinoembryonic antigen, human chorionic gonadotropin, serum and urine protein electrophoresis, fetal alpha protein were normal. Excisional biopsy of the submental lymph node was negative for malignancy. Wedge resection lung biopsy of the left upper lobe showed necrotizing granulomatous inflammation but no evidence of malignancy. Silver stain of the lung biopsy was suggestive of rare organisms like coccidioidomycosis. However, cultures of the lung tissue were negative for fungus and acid-fast bacilli. The cerebellar

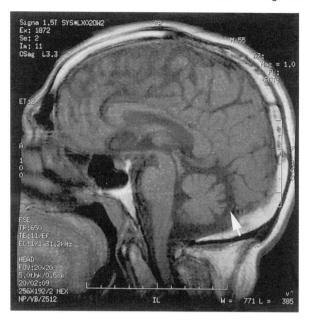

Fig. 24.1. A T1-weighted sequence MRI showing cerebellar atrophy.

ataxia did not improve despite thiamine therapy on admission. Furthermore, despite treatment with plasmapheresis and protein A immunoadsorption, the incapacitating cerebellar ataxia remained unchanged 6 months after the onset of symptoms. A diagnostic test was performed.

*   *   *

Discussion

The patient had a syndrome of acute and persistent bilateral cerebellar ataxia, transient ophthalmoparesis, and meningeal pleocytosis. The abducens paresis could have been due to the meningeal inflammation. Magnetic resonance imaging of the brain was non-revealing except for cerebellar atrophy. The chronic alcohol intake, ataxia, nystagmus and left abducens paresis raised the question of Wernicke syndrome but that was unlikely in the absence of an acute confusional state, the presence of CSF pleocytosis, and the lack of improvement with aggressive B1 vitamin treatment. The findings suggested an infection or inflammatory process. Human immunodeficiency virus (HIV) causes pathology of the central nervous system by direct invasion or by facilitating opportunistic infections such as progressive multifocal leukoencephalopathy, toxoplasma, syphilis, herpes, cytomegalovirus, and fungal infections. Acute meningitis associated with cranial neuropathies may develop at the time of seroconversion. Furthermore, HIV encephalitis manifests as a syndrome of cerebellar ataxia.[1-3] However, the patient's serum tested negative for HIV.

Cerebellar encephalitis, most commonly seen in children, is usually self-limited. Common causative agents include herpes zoster virus (HZV), mumps, measles, and rubella.[4] The clinical spectrum and infectious causes in adults are more varied than in children. In addition, whereas viral cerebellitis in young adults may be associated with good recovery, older patients are often left with permanent disability.[5] Causative agents in adults include HZV,[6] Epstein–Barr virus (EBV),[7,8] *Borrelia burgdorferi*,[9] syphilis, and *Mycoplasma pneumoniae*.[10] This patient had not traveled to endemic areas of Lyme disease and had no history of tick bite. The rare coccidioidomycosis-like structures seen on silver stain of the lung biopsy were difficult to interpret, especially in light of the negative cultures.[11] Furthermore, the absence of cerebellar abscesses and meningeal enhancement on MRI combined with the negative CSF cultures and stains for fungus argue against a fungal infection of the brain.[12]

Inflammatory conditions that cause cerebellar ataxia and meningeal pleocytosis include demyelination, vasculitis, and paraneoplastic cerebellar syndromes. The absence of white matter lesions on MRI of the brain argue against a demyelinating disease. The oligoclonal bands and elevated IgG synthesis rate in the CSF were nonspecific. Angiitis of the brain may be primary, or secondary to a systemic vasculitis or to an infection like syphilis, HZV, cytomegalovirus, HIV, mycoplasma and other bacterial, rickettsial, and fungal microorganisms, or any infection with excessive production of subarachnoid exudate.[13,14] Systemic vasculitides commonly associated with CNS angiitis include systemic lupus erythematosus,[15] Sjögren,[16] and Behçet syndromes.[17] The normal ESR and absence of stereotypical clinical features argue against systemic vasculitis. Angiitis of the brain is usually associated with white matter lesions on MRI, and cerebral angiography may show segmental narrowing of small blood vessels. Nonetheless, MRI of the brain and cerebral angiogram are often negative in vasculitis.[18,19] A biopsy is needed for diagnosis of angiitis of the brain.

The onset of paraneoplastic cerebellar ataxia is usually subacute but may also be abrupt.[20,21] Associated symptoms include ataxia, dysarthria, vertigo, diplopia, dysphagia, incoordination, oscillopsia, vertical or horizontal nystagmus, and dysmetria.[20,22] CSF may show transient lymphocytic pleocytosis, mildly elevated protein, elevated IgG synthesis, and oligoclonal bands.[20,22] Associated malignancies are ovarian cancer, breast cancer, lung cancer (small cell), lymphoma (Hodgkin disease), adenocarcinoma of unknown origin, and colon cancer. Nonetheless, it is predominantly associated with gynecological cancers; especially ovarian and breast,[23] and is rarely seen but has been reported in males.[4,24] The neurological symptoms usually precede the diagnosis of cancer, and the primary malignancy may never be found until autopsy.[20,22] The characteristic pathological findings are cerebellar atrophy, loss of Purkinje cells, thinning of the molecular and granular layers of the cerebellum, and there may be lymphocytic infiltrates in the leptomeninges, the dentate nucleus and the surrounding white matter. Imaging studies are usually nonspecific, and cerebellar atrophy may be present.[20,22] Serum and CSF may contain anti-Purkinje cell antibodies (APCA) that recognize multiple antigens expressed in Purkinje cells (Yo antigens). The predominant antigen, a 62 kDa protein, has been cloned and characterized.[25] The titer of the anti-Yo antibodies does not predict the course or the outcome of ataxia.[21,22,26,27] High dose steroids, intravenous immunoglobulin infusion, and plasmapheresis with or without protein A column adsorption have shown no proven efficacy.[27–29] Even after removal of the primary tumor, the patients with paraneoplastic ataxia may still be severely disabled by non-reversible cerebellar symptoms.

In summary, this clinical syndrome of acute cerebellar ataxia and lymphocytic meningeal pleocytosis in a 54-year-old male was consistent with either an infectious cerebellitis or a paraneoplastic cerebellar syndrome. We would test serum and CSF for anti-Yo antibodies, mycoplasma, HZV, EBV titers, and CSF for the genomes of HZV and EBV by polymerase chain reaction.

Serum ELISA for anti-Yo (APCA-1) antibodies was positive in a titer of 1:7680; Western blot analysis with Purkinje cell extracts was confirmatory. Repeat serum and CSF anti-Yo ELISA were also positive; the titers were 1:1920 and 1:512, respectively. ELISA analysis of the serum and CSF showed absence of anti-HU anti-RI antibodies (ANNA-1, ANNA-2).

The clinical course was consistent with idiopathic anti-Yo associated paraneoplastic cerebellar degeneration; no malignancy was found to data. The patient was to be followed closely and screened for malignancy at regular time intervals.

Diagnosis

Paraneoplasm.

References

1. McArthur JC. Neurologic manifestation of AIDS. *Medicine* 1987; **66**: 407–437.
2. Holland NR, Powers C, Mathews VP, Glass JD, Forman M, McArthur MB. Cytomegalovirus encephalitis in Acquired Immunodeficiency syndrome (AIDS). *Neurology* 1994; **44**: 507–514.
3. Atwood WJ, Berger JR, Kaderman R, Tornatore CS, Major EO. Human immunodeficiency virus type 1 infection of the brain. *Clin Microbiol Rev* 1993; **6**: 339–366.
4. Felician O, Renard JL, Vega F et al. Paraneoplastic cerebellar degeneration with anti-Yo antibody in a man. *Neurology* 1995; **45**: 1226–1227.

5. Klockgether T, Doller G, Wullner U, Petersen D, Dichgans J. Cerebellar encephalitis in adults. *J Neurol* 1993; **240:** 17–20.
6. Peters ACB, Verteeg J, Lindeman J, Bots GTAM. Varicella and acute cerebellar ataxia. *Arch Neurol* 1978; **35:** 769–771.
7. Lascelles RG, Longson M, Johnson PJ, Chiang A. Infectious mononucleosis presenting as acute cerebellar syndrome. *Lancet II* 1973; 707–709.
8. Gilbert JW, Culebras A. Cerebellitis in infectious mononucleosis. *JAMA* 1972; **220:** 727.
9. Neophytides A, Khan S, Louie E. Subacute cerebellitis in Lyme disease. *Int J Clin Pract* 1997; **51:** 523–524.
10. Komatsu H, Kuroki S, Shimizu Y, Takada H, Takeuchi Y. Mycoplasma pneumoniae meningoencephalitis and cerebellitis with antiganglioside antibodies. *Pediatr Neurol* 1988; **18:** 160–164.
11. Chitkara YK. Evaluation of cultures of percutaneous core needle biopsy specimens in the diagnosis of pulmonary nodules. *Am J Clin Pathol* 1997; **107:** 224–228.
12. Dunbar SA, Eason RA, Musher DM, Clarridge JE. Microscopic examination and broth culture of cerebrospinal fluid in diagnosis of meningitis. *J Clin Microbiol* 1998; **36:** 1617–1620.
13. Parisi JE, Moore PM. The role of biopsy in vasculitis of the central nervous system. *Semin Neurol* 1994; **14:** 341–348.
14. Landi G, Villani F, Anzalone N. Variable angiographic findings in patients with stroke and neurosyphilis. *Stroke* 1990; **21:** 333–338.
15. McNicholl JM, Glynn D, Mongey A, Hutchinson M, Bresnihan B. A prospective study of neurophysiologic, neurologic and immunologic abnormalities in systemic lupus erythematosus. *J Rheumatol* 1994; **21:** 1061–1066.
16. Alexander EL, Malinow K, Lejewski E, Jerdan MS, Porvost TT, Alexander GE. Primary Sjögren's syndrome with central nervous system disease mimicking multiple sclerosis. *Ann Int Med* 1986; **104:** 323–330.
17. Devlin TD, Gray L, Allen NB, Friedman AH, Tien R, Morgenlander JC. Neuro-Behcet's disease: factors hampering proper diagnosis. *Neurology* 1995; **45:** 1754–1757.
18. Ehsan T, Hasan S, Powers JM, Heiserman JE. Serail magnetic resonance imaging in isolated angiitis of the central nervous system. *Neurology* 1995; **45:** 1462–1465.
19. Alhalabi M, Moore PM. Serial angiography in isolated angiitis of the central nervous system. *Neurology* 1994; **44:** 1221–1226.
20. Peterson K, Rosenblum MK, Kotanides H, Posner JB. Paraneoplastic cerebellar degeneration. I. A clinical analysis of 55 anti-Yo antibody-positive patients. *Neurology* 1992; **42:** 1931–1937.
21. Hetzel DJ, Stanhope R, O'Neil B, Lennon VA. Gynecologic cancer in patients with subacute cerebellar degeneration predicted by anti-Purkinje cell antibodies and limited in metastatic volume. *Mayo Clin Proc* 1990; **65:** 1558–1563.
22. Posner JB. Paraneoplastic cerebellar degeneration. *Can J Neurol Sci* 1993; **20** (suppl. 3): 117–122.
23. Dropcho EJ. Autoimmune central nervous system paraneoplastic disorders: mechanisms, diagnosis, and therapeutic options. *Ann Neurol* 1995; **37:** S102–S113.

24. Krakauer J, Balmaceda C, Torres Gluck J, Posner JB, Fetell MR, Dalmau J. Anti-YO-associated paraneoplastic cerebellar degeneration in a man with adenocarcinoma of unknown origin. *Neurology* 1996; **46:** 1486–1487.

25. Fathallah-Shaykh H, Wolf S, Wong E, Posner JB, Furneaux HM. Cloning of a leucine-zipper protein recognized by the sera of patients with antibody-associated paraneoplastic cerebellar degeneration. *Proc Natl Acad Sci USA* 1991; **88:** 3451–3454.

26. Bolla L, Palmer RM. Paraneoplastic cerebellar degeneration. *Arch Intern Med* 1997; **157:** 1258–1262.

27. Graus F, Vega F, Delattre JY et al. Plasmapheresis and antineoplastic treatment in CNS paraneoplastic syndromes with antineuronal antibodies. *Neurology* 1992; **42:** 536–540.

28. Cher LM, Hochberg FH, Teruya I et al. Therapy for paraneoplastic neurologic syndromes in six patients with protein A column immunoadsorption. *Cancer* 1995; **75:** 1678–1683.

29. Ben David Y, Warner E, Levitan M, Sutton DMS, Malkin MG, Dalmau JO. Autoimmune paraneoplastic cerebellar degeneration in ovarian carcinoma patients treated with plasmapheresis and immunoglobulin. *Cancer* 1996; **78:** 2153–2156.

Case

25

A 26-year-old woman with fatigue and cramping of the foot

Clinical history and examination

A 26-year-old woman was referred for evaluation of a 5-year history of fatigue and cramping of her left foot.

Her birth and early developmental history were entirely normal. She was in good health and was employed as a registered nurse. At the age of 21, she experienced the onset of symptoms while working in nursing school. Initially she noticed that her left foot would feel fatigued after a busy day. At the age of 24 she was assigned to the 3:00 p.m. to 11:00 p.m. shift. She had no difficulty walking to work from the parking lot, however at the end of her shift she noticed that her left foot was inverted. She took 30 minutes to walk to her car after work. She compensated for this tendency by taping her left ankle in a position of extension so that it would not invert.

She noticed that the tendency of her leg to invert was worse after a poor night's sleep, after walking extended distances, after consumption of alcohol and at the beginning of her menstrual period. She also spontaneously reported that her leg never inverted in the morning. There was no history of weakness, numbness or parasthesias of the leg. There was also no history of neuroleptic or antiemetic exposure. Her family history was notable for her mother and for her sister who accompanied her to the office and are described below.

Neurologic examination revealed normal speech, comprehension and language. Cranial nerve examination revealed normal extraocular movements. There were no Kayser–Fleischer rings. There was also no facial masking or involuntary facial movements. Motor examination revealed full power and normal tone in the arms and legs. Her reflexes were 2+ and symmetric with down-going toes. Sensory examination was normal.

Coordination examination in the upper extremities was normal. When performing repeated foot-tapping with the left foot, her left ankle would stiffen and her toes would fan out. Continuing to tap her foot triggered inversion of the ankle. She walked with a normal stance and stride, however she recovered poorly on pull test, falling back into the examiner's arms.

The patient's 31-year-old sister and 54-year-old mother accompanied her to the office. Her sister was normal until the age of 6, when she developed a tendency to toe-walk, worse in the evening than the morning. She could regularly walk a half mile to school without difficulty, but was severely hampered by cramping of both feet and curling of her toes on her return trip. By the age of 12, her feet were constantly held in a flexed posture, and she underwent bilateral heel cord lengthening procedures which did not help. Her neurologic examination in the office was entirely normal except for inversion of the left foot which occurred when performing toe-tapping.

The patient's mother also developed similar symptoms at the age of 6. She was asymptomatic in the morning and gradually worsened throughout the day. Several years prior to evaluation, her gait became progressively slow and unsteady. Neurologic examination in the office revealed mild symmetric parkinsonism with cogwheeling and bradykinesia, worse in the legs than the arms. Inverted posturing of the feet was triggered by attempts to perform foot-tapping. Her gait was slow and mildly spastic and she recovered poorly on pull test.

No imaging studies were performed.

*   *   *

Discussion

This 26-year-old woman presents with a 5-year history of inversion of her left leg triggered by walking and foot-tapping. Her neurological examination was entirely normal except for her left foot movements. Her family history was remarkable for a sister and mother who evidenced a similar history and clinical profile, although more severe.

This patient's history and examination are striking. It would be very unusual for a primary neuromuscular disorder to present with inversion of one extremity. Similarly, central disorders of motor tone do not present in this fashion. The description of her symptoms and examination are highly suggestive of dystonia, and indeed this proved to be the correct diagnosis.

Dystonia is a syndrome best described as 'sustained muscle contractions that produce twisting and repetitive movements and abnormal postures.'[1] The term dystonia was first coined by Oppenheim in 1911 in his description of a disorder he called dystonia musculorum deformans, now known as DYT-1 dystonia.[2] Dystonia is a descriptive term – a patient may have dystonia, or features of their examination may be dystonic. Dystonia may be present when the patient is at rest, or it may appear when specific actions are performed, such as during writing. Dystonia that occurs exclusively during the performance of a specific task is termed task-specific dystonia.[3]

Dystonic symptoms may affect any part of the body. When they occur in one part of the body, such as in a limb or in the face or neck, dystonia is termed *focal*. When dystonia involves two adjacent body parts such as the face and neck, it is called *segmental*. Dystonia involving two or more noncontiguous areas is termed *multifocal*. *Generalized* dystonia refers to patients with dystonia in the legs who also have at least one other affected body area.[4]

Dystonia is a mysterious disorder, often intimidating even experienced clinicians. Part of the reason for this is that the number of conditions that can produce dystonia or dystonic features is very large. It is helpful to classify dystonia into four main categories using a system developed by Fahn (Table 25.1): primary dystonia (idiopathic), secondary dystonia, heredodegenerative dystonia (typically dystonia plus other neurologic disturbance), and dystonia-plus syndromes.[5]

Primary dystonia refers to disorders in which dystonia appears in isolation. Many patients with primary dystonia have an inherited form of the illness, and at last count there are more than 10 genetic loci responsible for dystonia. Only one gene for dystonia has been isolated; termed torsin A, it is an ATP-binding protein encoded on chromosome 9q. A single GAG deletion in this gene is responsible for most cases of childhood onset dystonia, originally called Oppenheims dystonia (and now known as DYT-1 dystonia). The disorder is autosomal dominant, but the penetrance is only 30–40%.[4]

The disorder usually begins at age 8–12, typically starting in a limb with task-specific dystonia (ankle inversion on walking, or writer's cramp). Patients who develop involvement of a leg tend to present earlier and progress more quickly. However, the rate of spread to other limbs is quite variable, as is the range of severity.[4] It is unknown whether or not adult-onset focal dystonia (for example blepharospasm, torticollis and writer's cramp) are genetic in origin.

Secondary dystonia, dystonia that occurs as the result of an injury or toxin exposure, is far more common than primary dystonia. Cerebral injury in the perinatal period may present with dystonia that accompanies spastic paresis, such as in cerebral palsy. Dystonia may also present months or even years after an injury has occurred, so-called delayed-onset dystonia. Head trauma, stroke, exposure to neuroleptics, and toxin exposure are other common causes of secondary dystonia.[5]

A number of heredodegenerative diseases present with dystonia in the company of other neurologic abnormalities. Among these conditions are X-linked dystonia–parkinsonism, seen primarily in the Filipino population,

Table 25.1. Etiologic classification of dystonia.

1. Primary (idiopathic) dystonia
   a. DYT-1 dystonia (Oppenheims dystonia)
   b. Adult-onset familial torticollis
   c. Familial cranial and limb dystonia (DYT-6)
   d. Sporadic, adult-onset, focal dystonia
2. Secondary dystonia
   a. Perinatal injury
   b. Postinfectious
   c. Head trauma
   d. Brain tumor
   e. Drug-induced (e.g. neuroleptic-induced)
   f. Toxins
3. Heredodegenerative diseases
   a. X-linked dystonia–parkinsonism (Lubag)
   b. Rapid-onset dystonia–parkinsonism
   c. Wilsons disease
   d. Niemann–Pick type C
   e. Juvenile neuronal ceroid-lipofuscinosis
   f. Hallervorden–Spatz
   g. Neuroacanthocytosis
4. Dystonia-plus syndromes
   a. Myoclonic dystonia
   b. Tyrosine hydroxylase deficiency
   c. Biopterin deficiency diseases
   d. Aromatic amino acid decarboxylase deficiency
   e. GTP cyclohydrolase I deficiency (dopa-responsive dystonia)

and autosomal dominant rapid-onset dystonia–parkinsonism. A variety of triplet repeat disorders may include dystonia in their presentation, including Huntingtons disease, Machado–Joseph disease and dentatorubro–pallidoluysian atrophy. Finally, many autosomal recessive disorders can present with dystonia, including Wilsons disease, Niemann–Pick type C, juvenile neuronal ceroid-lipofuscinosis, Hallervorden–Spatz disease and neuroacanthocytosis, among others.[5]

Dystonia-plus syndromes comprise the last category. These disorders present with dystonia with parkinsonism or myoclonus, and are not degenerative. Myoclonic dystonia is an autosomal dominant disorder in which patients develop myoclonus, dystonia or both. Usually beginning in the second decade, the condition is notable for its lightning-like jerks and exquisite response to alcohol. A number of disorders of the dopamine synthesis pathway may present with dystonia and parkinsonism. These include mutations in the tyrosine hydroxylase gene, disorders of biopterin and aromatic amino acid decarboxylase. Dopa-responsive dystonia, an autosomal dominant disorder of tetrahydrobiopterin synthesis, typically presents with dystonia and parkinsonism.

Diagnosis

The referring neurologist treated the patient with trihexyphenidyl, 1 mg twice a day. After 1 day of treatment, she reported no episodes of cramping of her foot at the end of the day. Her improvement was so dramatic that she was able to actively participate on a skiing trip without incident. Trihexyphenidyl was increased to 2 mg twice daily with resolution of symptoms in her leg, however she still complained of mild imbalance. Given the dramatic nature of her response, her sister was treated with trihexyphenidyl. She experienced dramatic benefit after taking 1 mg twice daily. Her mother also was treated with trihexyphenidyl with benefit in toe cramping, however her gait remained slow. Addition of Sinemet produced mild improvement in her symptoms.

Given the exquisite response to trihexyphenidyl, an oral phenylalanine loading test was performed on the patient, her sister and her mother (Fig. 25.1). This test confirmed that the patient and her sister had markedly impaired conversion of phenylalanine to tyrosine. Her mother's values were abnormal compared to a control patient with Parkinsons disease, although the abnormality was mild. This test confirmed the clinical suspicion of dopa-responsive dystonia, affecting the patient, her sister and her mother.

Dopa-responsive dystonia is an autosomal dominant disorder, first described in Japanese patients by Segawa et al.[6] It is a rare condition, with only several hundred cases reported in the world literature. Patients with dopa-responsive dystonia typically present in the first decade of life with gait disturbance, usually secondary to dystonia of the foot.[7] Children

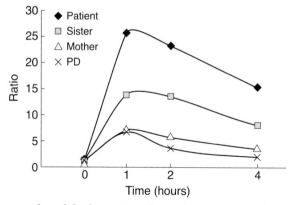

Fig. 25.1. Plasma phenylalanine to tyrosine ratios are shown for members of the family and for a control patient with Parkinsons disease (PD) after an oral load of phenylalanine. The patient and her sister show marked elevation of the ratio, indicating a reduction in the conversion of phenylalanine to tyrosine. The patient's mother's profile is only moderately abnormal compared to the control Parkinson patient.

eventually develop symptoms of parkinsonism, and the clinical picture can resemble cerebral palsy. Diurnal variation is a characteristic feature of the illness, although it is not universally present. When symptoms and signs reliably worsen in the evening and disappear in the morning, few other diagnostic possibilities exist.

Another characteristic feature is its exquisite response to levodopa. Symptoms and signs may completely disappear with low doses of levodopa, typically less than 300 mg per day. Anticholinergics like trihexyphenidyl are also highly effective in treating this condition. Unlike patients with Parkinsons disease, patients with dopa-responsive dystonia do not develop motor fluctuations, and the dose of levodopa can remain constant over time.[7] These characteristics mandate a therapeutic trial of levodopa in all children presenting with dystonia, in order to ensure that a diagnosis of dopa-responsive dystonia is not missed. The diagnosis should also be carefully considered in children who carry the diagnosis of cerebral palsy, particularly when there is no history of birth injury or when dystonic features are prominent.

Nygaard and colleagues[8] first mapped the gene for dopa-responsive dystonia to a region of chromosome 14q. The responsible gene was later identified by Ichinose, and the disorder was shown to be caused by mutations in the GTP cyclohydrolase I gene.[9] This enzyme catalyzes the first critical step in the synthesis of tetrahydrobiopterin. Deficiency in tetrahydrobiopterin leads to decreased tyrosine hydroxylase activity and a decrease in striatal dopamine. The penetrance of this condition is much higher in females than in males, although the reason for this difference is not known.[7] Also, the phenotypic spectrum of the disorder is wider than previously thought. Patients with dopa-responsive dystonia have been reported with adult-onset focal dystonia and adult-onset parkinsonism. The diagnosis should be considered in adult patients with Parkinsons disease who experience near-complete resolution of symptoms with low doses of levodopa for many years.

Given the variety of possible point mutations in the GTP-cyclohydrolase I gene, it is impractical to perform genetic analysis of an individual patient except in a research setting. Recently, interest has focused on the use of the oral phenylalanine loading test as a screen for dopa-responsive dystonia. In this test, subjects are given an oral load of phenylalanine, and blood samples are drawn over several hours to measure the conversion of phenylalanine to tyrosine. Symptomatic or asymptomatic carriers of the gene mutation have higher ratios of phenylalanine to tyrosine, due to inability to convert phenylalanine to tyrosine.[10] While this test is not foolproof, it can provide biochemical confirmation of the disorder. In this family, both sisters showed markedly abnormal ratios, and their mother's profile was also abnormal, although less severe. It is difficult to correlate the relative severity of her symptoms with her more benign biochemical defect.

This family's history illustrates the importance of securing a diagnosis of this eminently treatable condition. By considering the diagnosis, the treating physician can spare a patient the personal cost of living with a preventable disability.

Diagnosis

Dopa-responsive dystonia.

References

1. Fahn S. Concept and classification of dystonia. *Adv Neurol* 1988; **50:** 1–8.
2. Oppenheim H. Uber eine eigenartige Krampfkrankheit des kindlichen und jugendlichen Alters (Dysbasia lordotica progressiva, Dystonia musculorum deformans). *Neurol Centrabl* 1911; **30:** 1090–1107.
3. Tolosa ES, Marti MJ. Adult-onset idiopathic torsion dystonias. In: Watts RL, Koller WC, eds. *Movement Disorders*. New York: McGraw-Hill, 1997: 429–441.
4. Bressman SB, Fahn S. Childhood dystonia. In: Watts RL, Koller WC, eds. *Movement Disorders*. New York: McGraw-Hill, 1997: 419–428.
5. Fahn S. The classification of dystonia. In: *9th Annual Review of Movement Disorders*, 1999, unpublished.
6. Segawa M, Hosaka A, Miyagawa F et al. Hereditary progressive dystonia with marked diurnal fluctuation. In: Eldridge R, Fahn S, eds. *Advances in Neurology*, vol. 14. New York: Raven, 1976: 215–233.
7. Furukawa Y, Kish SJ. Dopa-responsive dystonia: recent advances and remaining issues to be addressed. *Mov Disord* 1999; **14:** 709–715.
8. Nygaard TG, Wilhelmsen KC, Risch NJ, et al. Linkage mapping of dopa-responsive dystonia (DRD) to chromosome 14Q. *Nat Genet* 1993; **5:** 386–391.
9. Ichinose H, Ohye T, Takahashi E. Hereditary progressive dystonia with marked diurnal fluctuation caused by mutations in the GTP cyclohydrolase I gene. *Nat Genet* 1994; **8:** 236–241.
10. Hyland K, Fryburg JS, Wilson WG et al. Oral phenylalanine loading in dopa-responsive dystonia: a possible diagnostic test. *Neurology* 1997; **48:** 1290–1297.

Refractory epilepsy

Clinical history and examination

A 32-year-old man was referred for further management of uncontrolled seizures.

He was in excellent health until age 15, when he had a head injury in a car accident. He lost consciousness briefly but recovered and was normal within 15 minutes. There were no residual neurological symptoms or signs. About 1 year later, he had a generalized tonic–clonic seizure. He had no premonitory symptoms ('aura') and only remembers awakening in a local emergency room.

Since age 16, he has averaged about one generalized tonic–clonic seizure per month. Observers have reported a sudden cry followed by stiffening of his entire body followed by shaking of the arms and legs; each episode lasts 1–2 minutes. He sometimes has urinary incontinence, and he has bitten his tongue on several occasions. He usually has no warning of a seizure, although on two or three occasions he has noted a strange sensation of whole body warmth immediately preceding the seizure. Similar symptoms have never occurred by themselves; he has not had staring spells.

In response to specific questioning, he described occasional brief muscle jerks of the arms, especially on the right, without other symptoms including alteration of consciousness. The jerks were most apt to occur in the morning and had become more frequent over the past few years; they were now occurring two or more times per week. Recently, he had also had a few generalized tonic–clonic seizures that had been preceded by a series of arm jerks.

There was no apparent diurnal pattern to his seizures, but he was convinced that seizures were more likely to occur during times of stress and when he was sleep deprived.

He was treated with phenytoin for 13 years, but he continued to have frequent seizures despite a maximal dosage of 400 mg/day, which produced stable plasma concentrations of 21 mg/dl. Three years ago, carbamazepine, 1500 mg/day, was substituted; blood levels averaged 10 mg/dl. This change did not result in improved seizure control, and he also reported excessive sleepiness and intermittent dizziness after starting carbamazepine.

There was no family history of epilepsy. Birth and developmental history were unremarkable, and there was no history of febrile seizures or brain infections.

Recent diagnostic testing included normal brain magnetic resonance imaging (MRI) and routine blood tests (complete blood count, serum chemistries, and liver function tests). An electro-encephalogram (EEG), recorded with the patient awake, was normal except for a single right-hemisphere spikewave discharge maximal in the frontal region. Hyperventilation and photic stimulation did not evoke abnormal potentials.

There was no relevant medical or surgical history. The only medication he was taking at the time of presentation was carbamazepine, 500 mg three times daily.

The patient had emigrated from the Dominican Republic 4 years ago. He had completed 2 years of college, but he was currently unemployed because of his epilepsy. There was no history of tobacco, alcohol, or substance abuse.

On physical examination, his temperature was 98.4F, the pulse was 72 beats/min, and the respiratory rate was 12/min. His blood pressure was 120/80. General physical examination was normal. There were no significant cutaneous abnormalities or body asymmetries.

Neurological examination was also normal. In particular, no abnormal movements were observed.

A diagnostic procedure was performed.

*   *   *

Discussion

The patient has a 16-year history of intractable epilepsy. Uncontrolled seizures should always lead to reconsideration of the diagnosis. In this case, there seems little question that the patient has epilepsy. Rather, the issue is the *type* of epilepsy. Stated another way, what *epileptic syndrome* does the patient have? Correct diagnosis or classification of a patient's epilepsy syndrome is important to optimal management, because this may affect critical treatment decisions. When confronted with a difficult case, it is always worth remembering a neurological fundamental truism: that careful analysis (or re-analysis, if necessary) is the cornerstone of accurate diagnosis.

In patients with epilepsy, it is first necessary to determine if the disorder is *localization-related* (that is, the seizures are of localized [partial] onset) or *generalized* (the seizures are generalized from the beginning).[1] In this patient's history, several features seem to point to a localization-related epilepsy whereas others indicate a generalized type of epilepsy. We will consider each of these in detail.

Localization-related epilepsies account for the majority of epileptic syndromes seen in adults: they represent about two-thirds of all cases.[2] Aspects of the history that suggest the seizures begin within a localized brain region include:

1. a head injury 1 year before onset of seizures;
2. rare prodromal symptoms (a feeling of body warmth);
3. arm jerking that was most pronounced on the right;
4. the epigastric sensation which preceded some of the seizures;
5. a lateralized EEG epileptiform discharge; and
6. the patient was from a developing country.

Auras are simple partial seizures characterized by stereotyped, subjective sensations unaccompanied by other, observable manifestations. Auras may occur in isolation or, most commonly, precede complex partial or generalized seizures. This sequence reflects propagation of the epileptic discharge from its point of origin to more distant brain regions. Auras are a hallmark of temporal lobe epilepsy but occur with other localization-related epilepsies as well. Common auras include an epigastric rising sensation, fear, a feeling of unreality or detachment, *déjà vu* and *jamais vu* experiences, metamorphopsia, and olfactory hallucinations. While this patient had had a sensation of warmth before, at most, three seizures, he had not had symptoms preceding the vast majority of seizures over 16 years. Furthermore, he never had similar symptoms independent of generalized seizures, and he had never had a complex partial seizure. Finally, the nature of this particular sensory experience is quite nonspecific and without the localizing value of the aforementioned examples. Given these considerations, it is unlikely that the warm feeling is an aura in the sense of being a specific epileptic event. It is more typical of a group of premonitory symptoms termed *epileptic prodromes*. These are inconsistent, nonspecific subjective feelings that occur minutes to a few hours in some patients before generalized tonic–clonic seizures. Among the more frequent sensations reported by patients are ill-defined anxiety, irritability, decreased concentration, and headache or other uncomfortable feelings.

What about the history of head injury? The association between head trauma and development of epilepsy has been recognized since antiquity.[3] However, the risk of developing epilepsy is related directly to the severity of the injury.[3] In a study of veterans of the Vietnam War who survived penetrating head injuries, the risk of developing epilepsy was increased 580-fold in the first year and remained 25-fold higher than baseline population rates after 10 years.[4] The risk associated with mild head injury is far less dramatic. In a large population-based study, mild head trauma (defined as loss of consciousness or memory for less than 30 minutes) increased the risk of epilepsy 1.5 times over control rates but only during the first 5 years following the injury.[3] Thereafter, the risk was similar to that in the general population. In the same study, the risk of post-traumatic seizures was increased three-fold in people with moderate head injuries and 17-fold in those with severe head injuries. Thus, the minor head injury sustained by this patient conveys only a slight increase in risk for developing epilepsy.

Another risk factor for localization-related epilepsy is the patient's origin in the Dominican Republic, a developing nation where he spent the first 28 years of his life. In developing nations, neurocysticercosis continues to be a major health problem because of poor sanitation. Infection of the central nervous system results after ingestion of the *Taenia solium* ova. In the brain, the parasites encyst and then typically degenerate over years until only small calcifications and associated gliosis remain. Occasionally degeneration of the cysts induces an intense inflammatory reaction that causes neurological deficits and acute symptomatic seizures. More commonly, the inactive calcified lesions result in symptomatic localization-related epilepsy. Both partial and secondarily generalized seizures occur in roughly equal proportions in affected populations.[5] Many studies have implicated neurocysticercosis as a major cause of epilepsy in developing nations; some have estimated that as many as 50% of chronic epilepsy cases are due to neurocysticercosis.[6] A critical review by Carpio et al.,[5] however, has pointed out that much of the data in the literature are unreliable and, consequently, the true risk is unknown. Although this risk may be overstated and its actual magnitude uncertain, neurocysticercosis increases the risk for localization-related epilepsy.

In this patient, the normal MRI scan excludes active parasitic infection but not inactive disease. The small punctate calcifications indicating old infection may not be well demonstrated by MRI. We do not have the results of a computed tomographic (CT) head scan, which is more sensitive to calcifications than MRI. Without any evidence of neurocysticercosis, it is impossible to say more than that his origin from a developing nation probably raises the risk of localization-related epilepsy by a small but unknown amount.

The EEG finding of a lateralized epileptiform discharge would seem to favor a localization-related epilepsy. However, this finding should be interpreted with caution. First, a single epileptiform event is often too small a sample to characterize adequately the pattern and clinical significance of the abnormality. Second, generalized discharges are not always fully elaborated; they can appear in partially developed forms. The frontal regions, especially, may reflect a 'focal' or lateralized expression of the abnormality.[7,8] Third, a sleep recording is often necessary to activate interictal, especially focal, epileptiform activity sufficiently for meaningful interpretation. In this case, the EEG finding is, in fact, ambiguous with respect to its favoring either a generalized or localization-related type of epilepsy.

Thus, there is actually only limited support for a diagnosis of localization-related epilepsy. In contrast, several aspects of the history offer stronger evidence for a generalized epileptic syndrome:

1. Seizures, despite their frequency, have always been generalized. There is no history suggesting partial seizures.
2. The muscle jerks are consistent with myoclonus,[9] and clusters of these had ended recently in generalized convulsions. Epileptic myoclonus is always an indication of a generalized, non-focal disorder. Electrographically, muscle jerks are associated with generalized bursts of spikes, polyspikes, and polyspike wave discharges. Myoclonic jerks can be fragmentary and asymmetric and, at any one time, predominate on one side of the body.
3. Phenytoin and carbamazepine were ineffective.

Myoclonic seizures occur in only a limited number of epilepsy syndromes. The various progressive myoclonic epilepsy disorders can be excluded given the patient's normal neurological examination 16 years after onset of symptoms, normal EEG background activity, and lack of family history.[10,11] Rather, this setting is typical of an idiopathic generalized epilepsy syndrome. Benign myoclonic epilepsy of infancy, myoclonic astatic epilepsy, epilepsy with myoclonic absences, and eyelid myoclonia with absences can all be excluded because of the age of onset, lack of drop attacks, and negative history for absence seizures.

The most reasonable diagnosis is juvenile myoclonic epilepsy (JME). The history contains several suggestive clues: onset of seizures in mid-adolescence; myoclonic jerks that occur predominantly in the morning; normal neurological history and examination; normal MRI scan; and an EEG abnormality that could be consistent with the diagnosis. Also consistent is the lack of response to antiepileptic drugs that are highly effective in partial and secondarily generalized seizures but typically ineffective in this syndrome.

Juvenile myoclonic epilepsy is the most common idiopathic generalized epilepsy syndrome: it comprises 4–6% of all types of epilepsy.[12–14] Most studies have found that males and females are affected equally.[15–17] Hereditary factors are clearly evident, and a family history of epilepsy can be obtained in 40–50% of patients.[12,15] In a population with a high rate of consanguinity, a positive family history was found in 66% of patients.[17] Several groups of investigators have reported linkage to chromosome 6p;[18] others have disputed this.[19,20] No gene has been found, and the mode of inheritance is unknown at present, although polygenic factors are likely.[21]

As its name indicates, this epilepsy syndrome begins in adolescence, usually between 12 and 18 years of age, but it can begin as early as 8 years or as late as 26 years.[13,15] Myoclonic seizures are present in all patients as they are required for diagnosis. They may be the only type of seizure in 2–10% of cases. Myoclonic jerks typically appear 2–3 years before generalized tonic–clonic seizures, although it is almost always the latter which bring the patient to medical attention. In most patients, 88% in one series,[17] myoclonic seizures occur shortly after awakening. This is especially marked in the setting of fatigue and sleep deprivation.[17] Myoclonic seizures can vary from small, arrhythmic, discrete muscle jerks to strong, bilaterally synchronous contractions of the arms and legs. Arm and hand muscles are most commonly affected, the trunk, neck, and legs less often.[15] Muscles of the face are usually not affected.[22] Occasionally the diaphragm is involved. When myoclonus is limited to the fingers, the patient may report clumsiness. Myoclonus of the legs results in falls. At times, the myoclonic seizure may consist entirely of a subjective internal shock-like sensation, without observable clinical signs.

A surprising proportion of patients report unilateral jerks. Panayiotopoulos et al.[17] described unilateral jerks in 23% of patients, most commonly on the right. Although handedness was not analyzed in this study, it may be that asymmetric jerks are more noticeable, and thus over-reported, in the dominant hand. When asymmetric, myoclonic jerks should not be mistaken for simple partial motor seizures.

Generalized tonic–clonic seizures occur in over 90% (range 79–98%) of patients with JME.[15,17,23] The tonic–clonic seizures also tend to occur within 1–2 hours of awakening, but the association is less pronounced than with the myoclonic seizures.[16,17] As in this case, the majority of patients report occasions when a crescendo of repetitive myoclonic jerks ends in a generalized tonic–clonic seizure.[15] Janz and Durner[16] have observed that the tonic–clonic seizures in JME are often violent with a prolonged tonic phase.

Absence seizures occur in about 35% (range 33–40%) of patients with JME.[15,17,23] They may be the first manifestation of the disorder, preceding the development of myoclonic jerks by several years.[12,17,24] Absences in JME are typically less frequent and less disruptive compared to childhood absence epilepsy (pyknolepsy).[16] As a result, absence seizures frequently go unnoticed in these patients.

Interictal EEG abnormalities in JME are characteristic of the disorder, but not pathognomonic.[15] Background activity is normal or near-normal. Epileptiform activity consists of generalized, bisynchronous spikes, spike wave, and polyspike wave discharges with a repetition rate of 3.5–6 Hz. The polyspike component is often evident only at the beginning of the spike wave paroxysm. With myoclonic jerks, the EEG shows bisynchronous brief runs of multiple spikes at frequencies of 10–16 Hz. The run of polyspikes is usually followed by bursts of high-voltage, irregular 2–5 Hz generalized slow waves with intermixed spikes. As in other idiopathic generalized epilepsy syndromes, many patients with JME also have bursts of rhythmic 2.5–3 Hz ('typical') generalized spike wave discharges.[15] A photoparoxysmal response is common, occurring in 27–41% of patients with JME.[7,13,17]

'Focal' EEG findings occur in up to 30–50% of patients with JME and other idiopathic generalized epilepsy syndromes.[7,8,17,25] To avoid misinterpretation, it is important to have criteria that help distinguish a partial or fragmentary expression of an underlying generalized abnormality from genuine focal spikes that indicate a localization-related epilepsy. Helpful features include the following:

1. In generalized epilepsy, 'focal' spikes are typically frontal (voltage maximal at F3 or F4).
2. The isolated spikes have morphologies similar or identical to that of spikes occurring as part of a generalized spike wave burst; they do not have the variable waveform exhibited by focal epileptogenic spikes.
3. Isolated spikes tend to shift from side to side; they do not repeat as in a localization-related epilepsy.
4. In patients with localization-related epilepsy, focal slowing in the same region as the spike abnormality is common. In generalized epilepsy, isolated spikes are not accompanied by focal slow waves.
5. In patients with generalized epilepsy, adequate recording always demonstrates that the predominant epileptiform abnormality is diffuse, bilateral and, for the most part, symmetric.

In this patient, a recent EEG had been interpreted as showing a 'focal' abnormality on the basis of a single frontal spike. Because the EEG findings have important implications for diagnosis and treatment, further recording should be done to obtain additional examples of the abnormality that will allow definitive characterization.

Diagnostic procedure

The patient was admitted to the epilepsy monitoring unit for continuous video–EEG recording. Carbamazepine was tapered and discontinued. Background EEG activity was always normal during both waking and sleep states. There were occasional 1–2 second bursts of generalized, bisynchronous 5–6 Hz spike wave and polyspike wave discharges that were expressed maximally over the frontal regions (Fig. 26.1). At times, the discharges were higher voltage on one side or the other (Fig. 26.2), but there was no persistent asymmetry. There was no photoparoxysmal response. Hyperventilation did not activate abnormalities.

Monitoring captured numerous myoclonic seizures, most of which occurred within 2 h of awakening. Clinically, these manifested as discrete, synchronous myoclonic jerks of varying intensity. The myoclonus mainly involved the arms but sometimes spread to the trunk. Muscle jerks were associated with brief bursts of generalized polyspike discharges (Fig. 26.3).

Valproate was started and the dosage titrated rapidly to 1500 mg/day. Within 72 hours, there was a significant decrease in the frequency of myoclonic jerks and number of spike wave bursts on EEG. Six months later, in a routine office visit, the patient had had no further generalized

0:23:16:26.00 10 sec 20 uV 1x 3 - Ref 0.1 sec 70 Hz 60 Hz

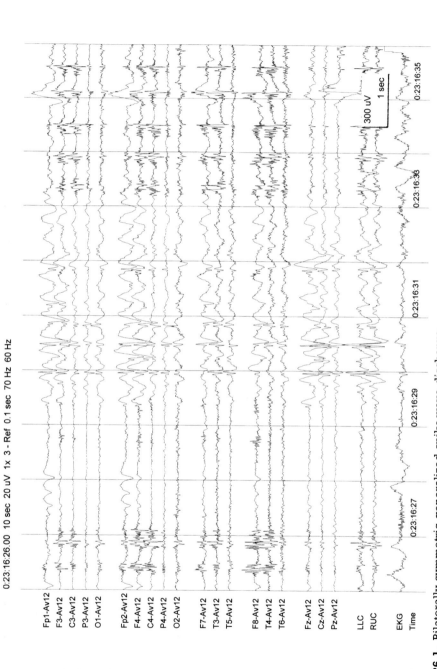

Fig. 26.1. Bilaterally symmetric generalized spike wave discharge.

0:00:05:20.00 10 sec 10 uV 1x 1 - BPlrlr 0.1 sec 70 Hz 60 Hz

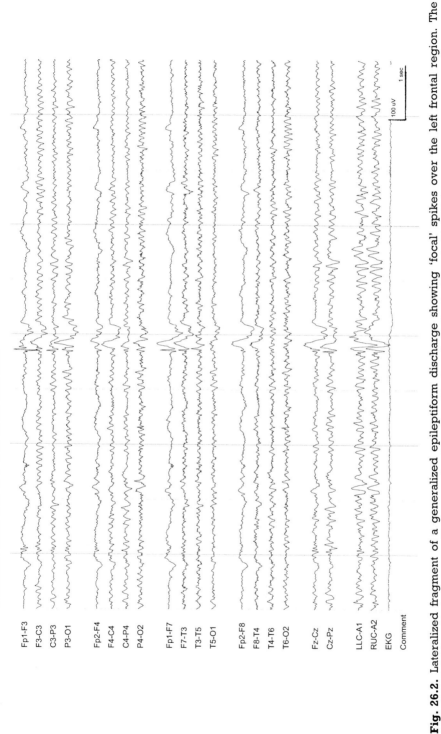

Fig. 26.2. Lateralized fragment of a generalized epileptiform discharge showing 'focal' spikes over the left frontal region. The majority of discharges in the recording were clearly generalized and similar to those in Fig. 26.1.

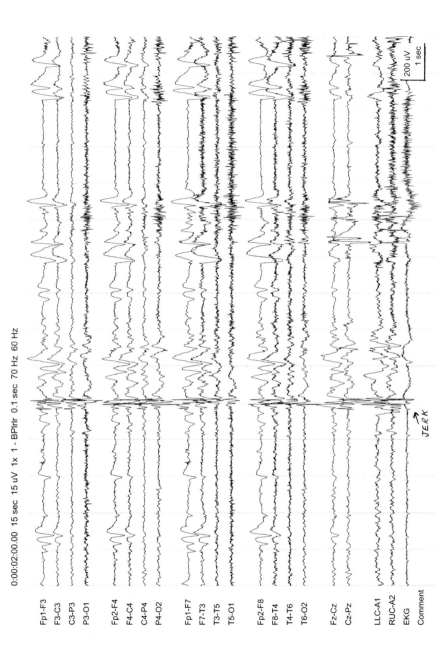

Fig. 26.3. Myoclonic seizure. Note that the myoclonic jerk is coincident with the burst of polyspikes which initiates the discharge.

tonic–clonic seizures and only two myoclonic seizures, both in the setting of sleep deprivation.

Further discussion

This patient illustrates several important practical issues. Although it is one of the most common epileptic disorders of adolescents and young adults, it is frequently misdiagnosed as in the patient discussed here. Several studies have found that delays in diagnosis average 8–15 years from onset of myoclonic seizures.[12,25,26] Several factors contribute to this. First, patients often do not recognize myoclonic jerks as a neurological symptom, especially when they are mild. Thus, myoclonus may not even be mentioned during a visit to the physician, and after the first tonic–clonic convulsion, physicians often fail to probe adequately for this characteristic feature. Worse, when myoclonic jerks are reported, patients and physicians alike frequently attribute them to nervousness, anxiety, and clumsiness. Thus, the defining symptom of JME is often neglected.

Two other factors that contribute to misdiagnosis have already been discussed: unilateral myoclonic jerks and 'focal' EEG abnormalities. As in this case, such findings seem to support a diagnosis of localization-related epilepsy, and treatment is instituted based on this assumption. When absence attacks are present, they are frequently misinterpreted as complex partial seizures.

The consequence of such faulty reasoning is reflected in the poor response to treatment. Phenytoin and carbamazepine are excellent drugs for localization-related epilepsies;[27] they are less effective against idiopathic generalized tonic–clonic seizures and may exacerbate myoclonic seizures[28–30] as seemed to happen in this patient after introduction of carbamazepine.

Several retrospective studies have shown valproate to be effective in treating all seizures types seen in JME. Valproate monotherapy controls seizures completely in about 85% (range 84–86%) of cases.[15,23,31] This is far superior compared to results seen in comparable studies of phenobarbital, primidone, and phenytoin.[16] For most patients, therefore, valproate is the drug of choice for JME, although growing experience with lamotrigine[32] and levetiracetam suggests that these drugs may be as effective and have fewer adverse effects. Controlled comparative trials are needed.

Physicians and patients have been concerned about two problems attributed to valproate: fatal hepatotoxicity and birth defects. In two thorough reviews, Dreifuss and colleagues[33,34] found no reports of fatal hepatotoxicity in patients older than 10 years who took valproate as monotherapy. Patients treated with valproate who developed fatal liver toxicity were children (most of them under 2 years of age) on polytherapy. The majority also had underlying medical illnesses, often inherited metabolic disorders. This issue, therefore, should be of little concern to patients with

JME, as the majority of affected individuals are healthy, older than 10 years of age, and require only the one drug.

With regard to use of valproate in women of childbearing age, the American Academy of Neurology has published useful consensus guidelines.[35,36] They conclude, first, that seizures themselves pose a significant risk to both mother and fetus, and therefore controlling seizures during pregnancy is a high priority. Second, there is no evidence that one antiepileptic drug is significantly better or worse in terms of risk. All increase the risk of major congenital malformations by two- to three-fold. Valproate has an additional 1–2% risk of neural tube defects, but this can be minimized by preconceptive use of folic acid in a dose of 1–2 mg/day.

Correct diagnosis is also necessary so that patients can be counseled appropriately about the need for lifestyle modifications and the necessity of long-term antiepileptic drug (AED) treatment. Patients must understand the need for regular sleep and that sleep deprivation almost invariably exacerbates myoclonus and generalized tonic–clonic seizures.[16,22,37] Alcohol consumption, too, is frequently associated with increased or breakthrough seizures and should therefore be eliminated or, at least, minimized.[22,23] Photosensitive patients should be advised to avoid circumstances in which flashing lights are likely to be encountered (e.g. discothèques). Patient education about the importance of complying with the prescribed drug regimen is another important aspect of treatment, because seizure relapse is common in the setting of missed doses of medication.

Patients should also know that long-term treatment is necessary in many patients because of a high rate of relapse, even after many years of being seizure-free, following planned drug withdrawal.

Diagnosis

Juvenile myoclonic epilipsy.

References

1. Commission on Classification and Terminology of the International League against Epilepsy. Proposal for revised classification of epilepsies and epileptic syndromes. *Epilepsia* 1989; **30:** 389–399.
2. Hauser WA, Kurland LT. The epidemiology of epilepsy in Rochester, Minnesota, 1935 through 1967. *Epilepsia* 1975; **16:** 1–66.
3. Annegers JF, Hauser WA, Coan SP et al. A population-based study of seizures after traumatic brain injuries. *N Engl J Med* 1998; **338:** 20–24.
4. Salazar AM, Jabbari B, Vance SC et al. Epilepsy after penetrating head injury. I. Clinical correlates: a report of the Vietnam Head Injury Study. *Neurology* 1985; **35:** 1406–1414.

5. Carpio A, Escobar A, Hauser WA. Cysticercosis and epilepsy: a critical review. *Epilepsia* 1998; **39:** 1025–1040.
6. Medina MT, Rosas E, Rubio-Donnadieu F et al. Neurocysticercosis as the main cause of late-onset epilepsy in Mexico. *Arch Intern Med* 1990; **150:** 325–327.
7. Aliberti V, Grunewald RA, Panayiotopoulos CP et al. Focal electroencephalographic abnormalities in juvenile myoclonic epilepsy. *Epilepsia* 1994; **35:** 297–301.
8. Lancman ME, Asconape JJ, Penry JK. Clinical and EEG asymmetries in juvenile myoclonic epilepsy. *Epilepsia* 1994; **35:** 302–306.
9. Janz D, Inoue Y, Seino M. Myoclonic seizures. In: Engel J, Pedley TA, eds. *Epilepsy: A Comprehensive Textbook.* Philadelphia: Lippincott-Raven, 1997; pp. 2389–2400.
10. Berkovic SF, Andermann F, Carpenter S, Wolfe LS. Progressive myoclonus epilepsies: specific cause and diagnosis. *N Engl J Med* 1986; **315:** 296–305.
11. Berkovic SF, So NF, Andermann F. Progressive myoclonus epilepsies: clinical and neurophysiological diagnosis. *J Clin Neurophysiol* 1991; **8:** 261–274.
12. Asconape J, Penry JK. Some clinical and EEG aspects of benign juvenile myoclonic epilepsy. *Epilepsia* 1984; **25:** 108–114.
13. Janz D. Epilepsy with impulsive petit mal (Juvenile myoclonic epilepsy). *Acta Neurol Scand* 1985; **72:** 449–459.
14. Murthy JMK, Yangala R, Srinivas M. The syndrome classification of the International League Against Epilepsy: a hospital-based study from South India. *Epilepsia* 1998; **39:** 48–54.
15. Delgado-Escueta AV, Enrile-Bacsal F. Juvenile myoclonic epilepsy of Janz. *Neurology* 1984; **34:** 285–294.
16. Janz D, Durner M. Juvenile myoclonic epilepsy. In: Engel J, Pedley TA, eds. *Epilepsy: A Comprehensive Textbook.* Philadelphia: Lippincott-Raven, 1997; pp. 2389–2400.
17. Panayiotopoulos CP, Obeid T, Tahan AR. Juvenile myoclonic epilepsy: a 5-year prospective study. *Epilepsia* 1994; **35:** 285–296.
18. Greenberg DA, Delgado-Escueta AV, Widelitz H et al. Juvenile myoclonic epilepsy (JME) may be linked to the BF and HLA loci on human chromosome 6. *Am J Genet* 1988; **31:** 184–192.
19. Elmslie FV, Williamson MP, Rees M et al. Linkage analysis of juvenile myoclonic epilepsy and microsatellite loci spanning 61 cM of human chromosome 6p in 19 nuclear pedigrees provides no evidence for a susceptibility locus in this region. *Am J Hum Genet* 1996; **59:** 653–663.
20. Whitehouse WP, Rees M, Curtis D et al. Linkage analysis of idiopathic generalized epilepsy and marker loci on chromosome 6p in families of patients with juvenile myoclonic epilepsy: no evidence for an epilepsy locus in the HLA region. *Am J Hum Genet* 1993; **53:** 652–662.
21. Durner M, Sander T, Greenberg DA et al. Localization of idiopathic generalized epilepsy on chromosome 6p in families of juvenile myoclonic epilepsy patients. *Neurology* 1991; **41:** 1651–1655.
22. Grunewald RA, Panayiotopoulos CP. Juvenile myoclonic epilepsy: a review. *Arch Neurol* 1993; **50:** 594–598.
23. Penry JK, Dean JC, Riela AR. Juvenile myoclonic epilepsy: long-term response to therapy. *Epilepsia* 1989; **30** (suppl. 4): S19–S23.

24. Panayiotopoulos CP, Obeid T, Waheed G. Absences in juvenile myoclonic epilepsy: a clinical and video-electroencephalographic study. *Ann Neurol* 1989; **25:** 391–397.

25. Grunewald RA, Chroni E, Panayiotopoulos CP. Delayed diagnosis of juvenile myoclonic epilepsy. *J Neurol Neurosurg Psychiatry* 1992; **55:** 497–499.

26. Panayiotopoulos CP, Tahan R, Obeid T. Juvenile myoclonic epilepsy: factors of error involved in the diagnosis and treatment. *Epilepsia* 1991; **32:** 672–676.

27. Mattson RH, Cramer JA, Collins JF et al. Comparison of carbamazepine, phenobarbital, phenytoin, and primidone in partial and secondarily generalized tonic–clonic seizures. *N Engl J Med* 1985; **313:** 145–151.

28. Lerman P. Seizures induced or aggravated by anticonvulsants. Epilepsia 1986; 27: 706–710.

29. Perucca E, Gram L, Avanzini G, Dulac O. Antiepilepic drugs as a cause of worsening seizures. *Epilepsia* 1998; **39:** 5–17.

30. Sozuer DT, Atakli D, Atay T et al. Evaluation of various antiepileptic drugs in juvenile myoclonic epilepsy. *Epilepsia* 1996; **37** (suppl. 4): 77.

31. Covanis A, Gupta AK, Jeavons PM. Sodium valproate: monotherapy and polytherapy. *Epilepsia* 1982; **23:** 693–720.

32. Timmings PL, Richens A. Efficacy of lamotrigine as monotherapy for juvenile myoclonic epilepsy: pilot study results. *Epilepsia* 1993; **34** (suppl. 2): 160.

33. Dreifuss FE, Langer DH, Moline KA et al. Valproic acid hepatic fatalities. II. US experience since 1984. *Neurology* 1989; **39:** 201–207.

34. Dreifuss FE, Santilli N, Langer DH et al. Valproic acid hepatic fatalities: a retrospective review. *Neurology* 1987; **37:** 379–385.

35. Delgado-Escueta AV, Janz D. Consensus guidelines: preconception counseling, management, and care of the pregnant woman with epilepsy. *Neurology* 1992; **42** (suppl. 5): 149–160.

36. Morrell MJ. Guidelines for the care of women with epilepsy. *Neurology* 1998; **51** (suppl. 4): S21–S27.

37. Pederson SB, Peterson KA. Juvenile myoclonic epilepsy: clinical and EEG features. *Acta Neurol Scand* 1998; **97:** 160–163.

Stroke

Clinical history and examination

Trying to get up from his chair a 69-year-old man fell to the ground with weakness of his right arm and leg. There was no headache, loss of consciousness, abnormal movement, visual or sensory symptoms, incontinence, chest pain, shortness of breath, or nausea. He lay on the floor for 3 hours thinking symptoms would clear; when they persisted he contacted the emergency medical service and was brought to the hospital.

He had had hypertension for many years, currently treated with amlodipine, enalapril, and metolazone. Three years earlier he had had a myocardial infarction, and cardiac catheterization at that time showed inferior and posterior septal akinesis and an occluded proximal right coronary artery with retrograde left-to-right flow through collaterals. Following the heart attack, he gave up what had been daily ethanol and tobacco use and intermittent cocaine use. His only other medication was isosorbide dinitrate.

In the emergency room blood pressure was 179/88 mmHg, pulse was 110/min and regular, respirations were 14 and regular, and temperature was 97.6°F. He was obese, but his general physical examination, including heart, lungs, and neck vessels, was normal. Except for a mild impairment in recent memory, mental status was normal, including verbal expression, speech comprehension, naming, and repetition. He had never learned to read and write. There was no apraxia and no hemineglect; pictures copied with his left hand were accurate. Speech was mildly slurred, and there was right-sided facial weakness which spared the forehead. The left pupil was 3 mm in diameter and the right 5 mm, and there was mild left ptosis. The right arm and leg were flaccid and paralyzed. There was very mildly decreased touch and pinprick sensation over his entire right side; other sensory modalities were normal. Tendon reflexes were 2+ and symmetric and there was a right extensor plantar response. Visual fields and eye movements were normal.

Hematocrit was 45%, hemoglobin 15.3/dl, white blood count 14 600/ mm^3 (87% polymorphonuclears, 9% lymphocytes, 3.6% monocytes, 0.2% eosinophils, and 0.2% basophils), platelets 269 000/mm^3, mean corpuscular volume 94 fl, and prothrombin time 11 seconds (INR 0.9). Blood glucose was 141 mg/dl; blood urea nitrogen, creatinine, sodium, potassium, chloride, carbon dioxide, calcium, phosphorus, bilirubin, albumin, globulin, aspartate aminotransferase, lactic dehydrogenase, uric acid, cholesterol, and creatine kinase were normal. Urinalysis was normal, and urine toxicology screening was negative for cocaine or other recreational drugs.

Chest radiography showed neither infiltrate nor cardiomegaly. Electrocardiography showed sinus tachycardia and Q waves in leads II, III, and aVF, but no acute ST-T wave changes.

A diagnostic study was performed.

*   *   *

Discussion

This man had several risk factors for stroke, namely hypertension, previous myocardial infarction, and a history of tobacco use. Sudden onset of focal symptoms and signs strongly suggests stroke even without such a background, and the presence of right-sided weakness involving the face, arm, and leg, in the absence of more than minimal sensory loss, language disturbance, or visual field defect, favors a small deep infarct affecting the corticospinal/corticobulbar tract at the level of either the internal capsule or the upper pons.[1-3] Infarction of the motor cortex in the frontal lobe could also cause weakness of face, arm, and leg, either by including the territories supplied by both the anterior and middle cerebral arteries or by occluding the middle cerebral artery proximally enough to damage the motor cortex as well as deeper corticospinal/corticobulbar projections. In either of these cases, it would be very unlikely that sensation, language, and visual fields would be spared.

The term *lacune* refers to a small deep infarct resulting from occlusion of a penetrating branch of a large cerebral or brainstem vessel. Such infarcts range from 0.2 to 15 mm^3 in diameter and affect territories supplied by vessels 100–400 µm in size.[4,5] They occur predominantly in the basal ganglia, internal capsule, thalamus, pons, and, less often, in white matter of cerebral gyri; they are rarely encountered in the cortical gray matter, corpus callosum, optic radiations, centrum semiovale, cerebellum, or medulla. A possible explanation for such distribution is that the affected small vessels, arising directly from large vessels, do not have gradual tapering of their diameters, rendering them susceptible to hypertensive and atherosclerotic damage. In addition, the territories supplied by these penetrators lack collateral blood supply.

Roughly three-fourths of patients with lacunes are hypertensive, and one-fourth are diabetic.[6,7] Vascular pathology includes microatheroma, lipohyalinois (reflecting chronic hypertension), and fibrinoid necrosis (reflecting more acute and severe hypertension). Infrequently, emboli are implicated.

Lacunar infarcts are less likely than large vessel atherostenotic infarcts to be preceded by transient ischemic attacks and more likely to progress over hours. Whether or not they produce symptoms depends on their size and location. Very small lacunes in the basal ganglia or thalamus may be asymptomatic; in fact, in a large autopsy study, only 19% of lacunes had produced symptoms.[8] A lacune involving the corticospinal/corticobulbar tract in the internal capsule or upper pons will cause 'pure motor stroke.'[3,9–14] (So will a lacune in the pyramidal tract of the medulla, but in that instance the face will be spared.[3,15]) A lacune involving the ventroposterior nucleus of the thalamus will cause 'pure sensory stroke.'[16–18] Less specific 'lacunar syndromes' include 'sensorimotor stroke' (affecting both the internal capsule and the thalamus),[19] 'stroke with ataxic hemiparesis' (affecting either the internal capsule or the basis pontis),[20–22] and 'dysarthria clumsy-hand syndrome' (affecting the anterior limb or genu of the internal capsule or the basis pontis).[23,24]

Seldom encountered today, perhaps because of effective treatment for hypertension, is 'lacunar state,' multiple bilateral lacunes producing episodes of hemiparesis superimposed on progressive gait difficulty, imbalance, pseudobulbar palsy, incontinence, and mental decline. The relation of lacunes to Binswangers disease or to vascular dementia is controversial; the presence of one or more lacunes in someone with progressive dementia hardly means that the dementia is vascular in origin.

In roughly 20% of patients with a so-called 'lacunar syndrome' another cause, either vascular or non-vascular, will be found.[8,25] In particular, if 'pure motor stroke' or 'pure sensory stroke' involve only two of three potential regions (e.g. face and arm but not leg; arm and leg but not face), cerebral cortex infarction and lacunar infarction are both reasonable possibilities. When a lesion is non-vascular, the specificity of the syndromes is even less; a frontal lobe neoplasm, for example, often causes only hemiparesis. Computed tomography (CT) excludes non-vascular syndromes such as neoplasm, abscess, and subdural or lobar intracerebral hematoma. Computed tomography detects lacunes in only 15–58% of cases, however, and, especially when performed within hours of onset, it can miss small cortical infarcts.[26,27] Magnetic resonance imaging detects lacunes in 74–98% of cases,[26,28] and diffusion-weighted MRI can be dramatically positive early in the course, confirming the acuteness of the lesion.

Results and clinical course

Computed tomography revealed a small deep infarct in the genu and anterior third of the posterior limb of the internal capsule (Fig. 27.1).

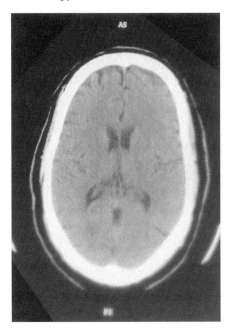

Fig. 27.1. Computed tomography scan showing a small area of lucency in the anterior part of the posterior limb of the left internal capsule, probably infarction. (Courtesy Dr Paoula Bowers.)

Magnetic resonance imaging with diffusion-weighted imaging (DWI) produced a strong signal in the same region (Fig. 27.2).

Antihypertensive medications were withheld, and he received aspirin 325 mg daily. There was steady improvement in his right hemiparesis; 2 days after admission his speech was only mildly slurred, flattening of the right nasolabial fold was the only evidence of facial weakness, and strength was normal in all limbs, with a right arm pronation drift and decreased rate and amplitude of rapid finger movements on the right. Sensation was normal except for mildly reduced cold sensation on his right limbs. He was fully oriented and could now recall three unrelated words after 5 min. He still had a left Horners syndrome, which, it was learned, had been present for at least 2 years. Carotid ultrasound examination showed mild intimal thickening of the common carotid arteries, but no plaques, stenosis, or evidence of dissection were apparent. Transesophageal echocardiography showed no thrombi or spontaneous echocontrast in the atria or ventricles, no diastolic dysfunction of the left ventricle, and a normal aorta. He was discharged 8 days after admission taking aspirin 325 mg daily plus his antihypertensive medications and isosorbide dinitrate; plans included CT of his chest to determine a possible cause of his Horners syndrome.

The corticospinal/corticobulbar tract enters the rostral internal capsule in the anterior half of the posterior limb and progressively shifts into the

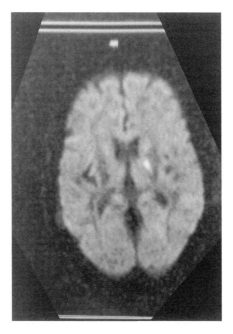

Fig. 27.2. Diusion-weighted MRI showing strong signal in the posterior limb of the internal capsule, probably signifying acute **Q2 infarction. (Courtesy Dr Paoula Bowers.)

posterior half of the posterior limb as it projects caudally.[29] The patient's lesion was thus in a predictable location. His improvement was also not surprising. In contrast to patients with a comparable degree of weakness following cerebral cortex infarction, patients with lacunes affecting the corticospinal tract usually improve, often rapidly and completely.[8,10,30] Although the prognosis is most favorable for partial hemiparesis, complete recovery is described in patients with complete hemiplegia.

Approximately 10% of patients with lacunar infarcts have a recurrent stroke within a year, with a similar rate of recurrence in subsequent years.[31,32] Only about one-fourth of recurrent strokes are lacunar, and they are more likely to occur in hypertensive patients.[33]

Diagnosis

Small deep infarct in the posterior limb of the left internal capsule.

References

1. Fisher CM. Lacunes: small deep cerebral infarcts. *Neurology* 1965; **15:** 774–784.

2. Fisher CM. Lacunar strokes and infarcts: a review. *Neurology* 1982; **32:** 871–876.
3. Fisher CM, Curry HB. Pure motor hemiplegia of vascular origin. *Arch Neurol* 1965; **13:** 130–140.
4. Fisher CM. Capsular infarcts. *Arch Neurol* 1979; **36:** 65–73.
5. Fisher CM. The arterial lesions underlying lacunes. *Acta Neuropathol* 1969; **12:** 1–15.
6. Mohr JP, Caplan LR, Melski JW et al. The Harvard Cooperative Stroke Registry. *Neurology* 1978; **28:** 754–762.
7. Mast H, Thompson JL, Lee SH et al. Hypertension and diabetes mellitus as determinants of multiple lacunar infarcts. *Stroke* 1995; **26:** 30–33.
8. Mohr JP, Marti-Vilalta J-L. Lacunes. In: Barnett HJM, Mohr JP, Stein B, Yatsu F, eds. *Stroke: Pathophysiology, Diagnosis, and Management*, 3rd edn. New York: Churchill Livingstone, 1999: 599–622.
9. Fisher CM, Caplan LR: Basilar artery branch occlusion: a cause of pontine infarction. *Neurology* 1971; **21:** 900–905.
10. Rascol A, Clanet M, Manelfe C et al. Pure motor hemiplegia: CT study of 30 cases. *Stroke* 1982; **13:** 11–17.
11. Reimers J, deWytt C, Seneviratne B. Lacunar infarction: a 12 month study. *Clin Exp Neurol* 1987; **24:** 27–32.
12. Richter RW, Brust JCM, Bruun B, Shafer SQ. Frequency and course of pure motor hemiparesis: a clinical study. *Stroke* 1977; **8:** 58–60.
13. Tuszynski MH, Petito CK, Levy DE. Risk factors and clinical manifestations of pathologically verified lacunar infarctions. *Stroke* 1989; **20:** 990–999.
14. Arboix A, Marti-Vilalta JL, Garcia JH. Clinical study of 227 patients with lacunar infarcts. *Stroke* 1990; **21:** 842–847.
15. Chokroverty S, Rubino FA, Haller C. Pure motor hemiplegia due to pyramidal infarction. *Arch Neurol* 1975; **2:** 647–648.
16. Fisher CM. Pure sensory stroke involving face, arm, and leg. *Neurology* 1965; **15:** 76–80.
17. Fisher CM. Thalamic pure sensory stroke: a pathologic study. *Neurology* 1978; **28:** 1141–1144.
18. Fisher CM. Pure sensory stroke and allied conditions. Stroke 1982; **13:** 434–437.
19. Mohr JP, Kase CS, Meckler RJ, Fisher CM. Sensorimotor stroke. *Arch Neurol* 1977; **34:** 739–741.
20. Fisher CM. Homolateral ataxia and crural paresis. A vascular syndrome. *J Neurol Neurosurg Psychiatry* 1965; **28:** 48–55.
21. Fisher CM. Ataxic hemiparesis. *Arch Neurol* 1978; **35:** 126–128.
22. Huang CY, Lui FS. Ataxic hemiparesis: localization and clinical features. *Stroke* 1984; **15:** 363–366.
23. Fisher CM. A lacunar stroke: the dysarthria clumsy hand syndrome. *Neurology* 1967; **17:** 614–617.
24. Spertell RB, Ransom BR. Dysarthria clumsy hand syndrome produced by capsular infarct. *Ann Neurol* 1979; **6:** 263–265.
25. Madden KP, Karanja PN, Adams HP et al. Accuracy of initial stroke subtype diagnosis in the TOAST study. *Neurology* 1995; **45:** 1975–1979.
26. Salgado ED, Weinstein M, Furlan AF et al. Proton magnetic resonance imaging in cerebrovascular disease. *Ann Neurol* 1986; **20:** 502–507.

27. Brown MM, Hesselink JR, Rothrock JF. MR and CT of lacunar infarcts. *AJNR* 1988; **9:** 477–482.
28. Rothrock JF, Lyden PD, Hesselink JR et al. Brain magnetic resonance imaging in the evaluation of lacunar infarcts. *Stroke* 1987; **18:** 781–786.
29. Ross ED. Localization of the pyramidal tract in the internal capsule by whole brain dissection. *Neurology* 1980; **30:** 59–64.
30. Pullicino P, Nelson RF, Kendall BE, Marshall J. Small deep infarcts diagnosed on computed tomography. *Neurology* 1980; **30:** 1090–1096.
31. Hier DB, Foulkes MA, Swiontoniowski M et al. Stroke recurrence within 2 years after ischemic infarction. *Stroke* 1991; **22:** 155–161.
32. Sacco SE, Whisnant JP, Broderick J et al. Epidemiological characteristics of lacunar infarcts in a population. *Stroke* 1991; **22:** 1236–1241.
33. Clavier I, Hommel M, Besson G et al. Long-term prognosis of symptomatic lacunar infarcts. A hospital-based study. *Stroke* 1995; **25:** 2005–2009.

Asymmetric muscle weakness

Clinical history and examination

A 40-year-old lawyer complained of pain in both shoulders, right more than left.

She had noticed a pain in the shoulders intermittently for at least 10 years, but this was becoming more troublesome, and she was now finding it increasingly difficult to lift her arms to clean her teeth, to brush her hair, and adjust her lawyer's wig. She had not noticed any other difficulty in the arms, and had no symptoms in the legs.

The medical history was otherwise not relevant to the current disorder. She had two sons aged 6 and 8 years who were well. There was no family history of neurologic disease.

Her temperature was 37.1°C, pulse 68, and respirations 15 per minute. The blood pressure was 120/85.

On physical examination, she had mild wasting and weakness of the shoulder girdle muscles, especially of trapezius, more marked on the right than the left. Power in the other muscles of the upper and lower limbs was normal. Tone, coordination and sensation were normal. Reflexes were normal and symmetrical, with bilateral flexor plantar responses. There was mild facial asymmetry, and retinal changes, with a small number of perimacular exudates. The cranial nerve examination was otherwise normal.

The urine was normal. Hematologic laboratory findings were normal, including normal hematocrit, hemoglobin, white cell count, platelet count, and ESR (6 mm/h). Blood chemical findings included normal sodium, potassium, and liver enzymes. Nonfasting glucose was mildly raised (8 mmol/l). Creatine kinase was mildly raised at 350 IU/l (normal < 100 IU/l).

Nerve conduction studies demonstrated normal motor and sensory conduction in the upper and lower limbs. Electromyography of the right trapezius demonstrated no spontaneous activity. The interference pattern was full, with a moderate number of low amplitude, short duration, polyphasic potentials. There were occasional additional high amplitude polyphasic potentials, but otherwise normal units. Similar findings were present in left biceps. Electromyography of right quadriceps femoris was normal. Muscle biopsy of right biceps was abnormal. There was variation in fiber size, with diameters ranging from 30 to 110 microns, including small angular fibers. Some 'moth eaten' fibers were seen. Inflammatory cells were present in the epimysium, but not within fibers. No ragged red fibers were seen. ATPase showed a normal fiber type distribution. Enzymatic studies were otherwise normal. A diagnostic test was performed.

*   *   *

Discussion

This 40-year-old woman presented with nonspecific pain in the shoulders, with additional weakness in the shoulder girdle. The differential diagnosis includes a myopathic, neuropathic, or arthritic process. The preserved reflexes, preserved sensation, and EMG findings, point to a primary myopathic process, which is confirmed further by the findings on muscle biopsy of the clinically unaffected right biceps. The myopathy could be either an intrinsic condition, i.e. a muscular dystrophy, or an inflammatory condition, i.e. a myositis. The long course of the condition makes a muscular dystrophy most likely. Inflammatory changes may be a nonspecific finding in muscle biopsies of patients with muscular dystrophies.

The clinical presentation of the muscular dystrophy is in a limb girdle distribution, affecting the shoulder girdle only. The underlying molecular and protein abnormalities in the limb girdle muscular dystrophies (LGMD) is becoming clearer, and it is now possible to define some of these (Table 28.1).[1,2] The proteins involved are constituents of the dystrophin-associated complex which includes the sarcoglycans, dystroglycans, and syntrophin. The sarcoglycans and dystroglycans are transmembrane proteins. They span the sarcolemma, interacting with dystrophin within, and laminin in the extracellular matrix. The protein abnormality may be sought by immunocytochemistry on the muscle biopsy, and should include dystrophin (which may be abnormal in sarcoglycanopathy), a range of sarcoglycan antibodies, and dysferlin. Calpain 3 currently requires immunoblotting. These were all normal in this patient.

In the absence of a family history, an autosomal recessive muscular dystrophy, a *de novo* dominant mutation, incomplete clinical penetrance of an autosomal dominant mutation, a manifesting female carrier of an X-linked muscular dystrophy, or nonpaternity, should be considered. Additional mild facial asymmetry was noted. This would extend the

Table 28.1. Genetic classification of limb girdle muscular dystrophies.

	Gene	Gene locus	Gene product
Autosomal dominant LGMD	LGMD1A	5q22-24	?
	LGMD1B	1q11-1	?
	LGMD1C	3p25	caveolin 3 (CAV3)
Autosomal recessive LGMD			
Calpain deficient LGMD	LGMD2A	15q15.1-21.2	calpain 3 (CAPN3)
Dysferlin deficient LGMD	LGMD2B	2p13	dysferlin (DYSF)
	LGMD2G	17q11-12	telethonin
	LGMD2H	9q31-33	?
Sarcoglycanopathies			
α-sarcoglycanopathy	LGMD2D	17q12-21.33	α-sarcoglycan (adhalin)
β-sarcoglycanopathy	LGMD2E	4q12	β-sarcoglycan (SGCB)
γ-sarcoglycanopathy	LGMD2C	13q13	γ-sarcoglycan (SGCG)
δ-sarcoglycanopathy	LGMD2F	5q33-34	δ-sarcoglycan (SGCD)

Based on Bushby 1999.[2]
? = gene and product unknown at present.

differential diagnosis to include facioscapulohumeral dystrophy (FSHD).[3,4] As an isolated case, facial weakness may be minimal, often manifesting with mild facial asymmetry and, for example, difficulty in whistling. The condition is slowly progressive, and whilst with careful examination up to 95% of those carrying the genetic abnormality will have clinical features at age 20 years,[5] the patient and family may not be aware of these features. Presentation with pain in the shoulder girdle may be related to musculoskeletal strain secondary to mild weakness.

A retinal abnormality is a recognized association of FSHD.[4] The characteristic features are of Coats' disease, with an abnormal retinal lipid exudate, due to leakage from the damaged epithelial cells of small retinal blood vessels. Fluoroscein angiography has demonstrated telangiectatic retinal vessels in 75% of patients with FSHD.[6] Most patients have no visual symptoms, but rare patients may have sight-threatening exudates. Photocoagulation of the telangiectatic vessels may prevent this. The characteristic appearance is a perimacular circinate distribution of exudates. Clinical hearing abnormalities are rare in patients with FSHD, but most patients have subclinical hearing impairment.[7]

Biochemical findings are often normal, although creatine kinase may be variably raised. Electromyography will generally show myopathic changes, although features more commonly associated with a neuropathic process, including large amplitude polyphasic potentials may also be found. Muscle biopsy may be normal, or show nonspecific myopathic features. Variable degrees of inflammatory change are recognized,[8] but these may also be found in other muscular dystrophies, including Duchenne muscular dystrophy.

Table 28.2. Diagnostic criteria for facioscapulohumeral dystrophy (FSHD).

Inclusion

Weakness of face or scapular stabilizers (in familial cases, facial weakness is present in >90% of affected individuals)

Scapular stabilizer weakness greater than hip–girdle weakness (applicable in mild to moderate FSHD)

Autosomal dominant inheritance in familial cases

Exclusion

Extraocular or pharyngeal muscle weakness

Prominent and diffuse elbow contractures

Cardiomyopathy

Distal symmetric sensory loss

Dermatomyositic rash or signs of an alternative diagnosis

Electromyographic evidence of myotonia or neurogenic potentials

Supportive features

Asymmetry of muscle weakness

Descending sequence of involvement

Early, often partial, abdominal muscle weakness (positive Beevor sign)

Sparing of deltoid muscles

Typical shoulder profile: straight clavicles, forward sloping of shoulders

Relative sparing of neck flexors

Selective weakness of wrist extensors in distal upper extremities

Sparing of calf muscles

High-frequency hearing loss

Retinal vasculopathy

Produced by the Facioscapulohumeral Consortium at the International Conference on the Cause and Treatment of FSHD, Boston, 1997 (Tawil et al.[9]).

The clinical features found in FSHD are shown in Table 28.2.[9] The differential diagnosis includes desmin myopathy, polymyositis, inclusion body myositis, mitochondrial myopathy, and congenital myopathies. Limb girdle dystrophies and scapuloperoneal myopathies may cause particular difficulty in clinical distinction, as they may have mild facial weakness. Sporadic cases of these disorders may be impossible to distinguish from FSHD on clinical and histologic criteria.

Further investigation and management

Blood was taken for DNA analysis. When the DNA was digested with the restriction site enzyme EcoRI, the p13E11 labeled fragment separated using pulsed field gel electrophoresis measured 31 kb. Double digestion with EcoRI and BlnI showed a small reduction in the fragment size to 28 kb. In patients with FSHD the EcoRI fragment is generally less than 38 kb, and in normal individuals greater than 41 kb.[10]

Facioscapulohumeral dystrophy is an autosomal dominant inherited muscular dystrophy. The gene for FSHD is on chromosome 4q, in the telomeric region.[11] Approximately 30% of individuals with FSHD have a *de novo* mutation,[10,12] and germ line mosaicism may account for other patients without a preceding family history.[13] The genetic abnormality is a reduction in the number of large (3.3 kb) repeat DNA sequences, termed D4Z4.[14] It is this reduction in the number of repeats which is measured in the genetic 'test.' Similar D4Z4 repeats are also present on chromosome 10q, and it is the digestion with both EcoRI and BlnI which allows these two similar sequences to be distinguished.[15] The repeats on chromosome 10q are digested by EcoRI, whilst those on chromosome 4q are not, allowing the 4q (FSHD) fragment (labeled with p13E11 probe) to be sized using pulsed field gel electrophoresis. (There is a single BlnI restriction site on the proximal portion of the chromosome 4q EcoRI fragment proximal to the D4Z4 repeats, leading to a small reduction in size of this fragment by approximately 3 kb.[3,15]) Further complications in molecular diagnosis include exchange of D4Z4 repeats between chromosomes 4q and 10q.[16] The mechanism by which the reduced number of D4Z4 repeats causes the disease, including the protein(s) involved, remains unknown at present.

There is an association between the number of repeats and severity of disease, with milder forms tending to have larger sizes (as in this patient).[17,18] The repeat size is stable from generation to generation, and the anticipation observed with dynamic short trinucleotide repeats, such as in myotonic dystrophy, is not observed. Careful study of patients with FSHD has suggested a mild degree of clinical anticipation, but there is no molecular explanation for this.[18]

Facioscapulohumeral dystrophy is the third most common muscular dystrophy, after Duchenne muscular dystrophy and myotonic dystrophy. The prevalence is approximately 4 per 100 000. The clinical features are shown in Table 28.2.[9] Age at onset is from infancy to middle age. The extent of muscle involvement among patients is variable and may range from minimal facial weakness to disability requiring a wheelchair, which eventually occurs in approximately 20% of patients. Lifespan is not significantly affected.[17]

There is no specific curative treatment for FSHD.[3] Treatment with steroids, suggested by the presence of inflammatory changes on muscle biopsy, has not proven to be effective.[19] A pilot study of albuterol, a beta-agonist, has suggested some mild benefit,[20] and a larger study of this medication is currently in progress. Other treatments to be considered include physiotherapy, and appropriate aids and appliances. Surgical scapular fixation may have some benefit in improving arm elevation, but fixation is difficult and the scapula may work loose.[21] Gold weights have been used to correct the difficulty in eye closure, and prevent exposure keratitis.[22]

Diagnosis

Facioscapulohumeral dystrophy (FSHD).

References

1. Molnar MJ, Karpati G. Muscular dystrophies related to deficiency of sarco-lemmal proteins. In: Schapira AHV, Griggs RC. *Muscle Diseases*. Boston: Butterworth-Heinemann, 1999: 83–114.
2. Bushby KMD. Making sense of the limb-girdle muscular dystrophies. *Brain* 1999; **122:** 1403–1420.
3. Orrell RW, Griggs RC. Muscular dystrophies: overview of clinical and molecular approaches. In: Schapira AHV, Griggs RC, eds. *Muscle Diseases*. Boston: Butterworth-Heinemann, 1999: 59–82.
4. Fitzsimons RB. Facioscapulohumeral muscular dystrophy. *Curr Opin Neurology* 1999; **12:** 501–511.
5. Lunt P, Compston DAS, Harper PS. Estimation of age dependent penetrance in facioscapulohumeral muscular dystrophy by minimising ascertainment bias. *J Med Genet* 1989; **26:** 755–760.
6. Fitzsimons RB, Gurwin EB, Bird AC. Retinal vascular abnormalities in facio-scapulohumeral muscular dystrophy: a general association with genetic and therapeutic implications. *Brain* 1987; **110:** 631–648.
7. Brouwer OF, Padberg GW, Ruys CJM et al. Hearing loss in facioscapulohum-eral muscular dystrophy. *Neurology* 1991; **41:** 1878–1881.
8. Arahata K, Ishihara T, Fukunaga H et al. Inflammatory response in faciosca-pulohumeral muscular dystrophy (FSHD): immunocytochemical and genetic analyses. *Muscle Nerve* 1995; (suppl. 2): S56–S66.
9. Tawil R, Figlewicz DA, Griggs RC et al. Facioscapulohumeral muscular dystrophy: a distinct regional myopathy with a novel molecular pathogenesis. *Ann Neurol* 1998; **43:** 279–282.
10. Orrell RW, Tawil R, Forrester J et al. Definitive diagnosis of facioscapulo-humeral dystrophy. *Neurology* 1999; **153:** 1822–1826.
11. Wijmenga C, Frants RR, Brouwer OF et al. Location of facioscapulohumeral muscular dystrophy gene on chromosome 4. *Lancet* 1990; **336:** 651–653.
12. Zatz M, Marie SK, Passos-Bueno MR et al. High proportion of new mutations and possible anticipation in Brazilian facioscapulohumeral muscular dystrophy families. *Am J Hum Genet* 1995; **56:** 99–105.
13. Griggs RC, Tawil R, Storvick D et al. Genetics of facioscapulohumeral muscular dystrophy: new mutations in sporadic cases. *Neurology* 1993; **43:** 2369–2372.
14. Van Deutekom JCT, Wijmenta C, van Tienhoven EAE et al. FSHD associated DNA rearrangements are due to deletions of integral copies of a 3.2 kb tandemly repeated unit. *Hum Mol Genet* 1993; **2:** 2037–2042.
15. Deidda G, Cacurri S, Piazzo N, Felicetti L. Direct detection of 4q35 rearrange-ments implicated in facioscapulohumeral muscular dystrophy (FSHD). J Med Genet 1996; **33:** 361–365.
16. Van Deutekom JCT, Bakker E, Lemmers RJLF et al. Evidence for subtelo-meric exchange of 3.3 kb tandemly repeated units between chromosomes 4q35 and 10q26: implications for genetic counselling and etiology of FSHD1. *Hum Mol Genet* 1996; **5:** 1997–2003.

17. Lunt PW, Jardine PE, Koch MC et al. Correlation between fragment size at D4F104S1 and age at onset or at wheelchair use, with a possible generational effect, accounts for much phenotypic variation in 4q35 facioscapulohumeral muscular dystrophy (FSHD). *Hum Mol Genet* 1995; **4:** 951–958.

18. Tawil R, Forrester J, Griggs RC et al. Evidence for anticipation and association of deletion size with severity in facioscapulohumeral muscular dystrophy. *Ann Neurol* 1996; **39:** 744–748.

19. Tawil R, McDermott MP, Pandya S et al. A pilot trial of prednisone in facioscapulohumeral muscular dystrophy. *Neurology* 1997; **48:** 46–49.

20. Kissel JT, McDermott MP, Natarajan R et al. Pilot trial of albuterol in facioscapulohumeral dystrophy. *Neurology* 1998; **50:** 1402–1406.

21. Bunch WH, Siegel IM. Scapulothoracic arthrodesis in facioscapulohumeral muscular dystrophy. Review of seventeen procedures with three to twenty-one year follow-up. *J Bone Joint Surg* 1993; **75A:** 372–376.

22. Sansone V, Boynton J, Palenski C. Use of gold weights to correct lagophthalmos in neuromuscular disease. *Neurology* 1997; **48:** 1500–1503.

Complex familial neuropathy

A 39-year-old, right-handed woman was admitted to the hospital because of worsening muscle weakness and sensory disturbance in her hands.

The patient had never been keen to participate in sports at school. Deformities of both feet had been noted in childhood. She had first come to the attention of neurologists 15 years previously with subacute progression of lower limb muscle weakness, over a 3-month period, associated with tingling in her feet. Her gait had continued to deteriorate, albeit more slowly, and she required surgery to both feet 7 years before the current presentation. She also began to wear ankle–foot orthoses at that time. She became aware of the worsening muscle weakness of her hands 1 month before hospital admission. Simultaneously, both hands became increasingly numb and started to tingle. She had difficulty holding a cup or a pen. There was no history of neck or back pain, nor of disturbance of sphincter control.

Her previous medical history was otherwise remarkable for a diagnosis of ulcerative colitis, 5 years before admission, lately in remission.

Several members of her family also had deformities of the feet and an abnormal gait (Fig. 29.1).

The patient worked as a teacher. She was a non-smoker and drank little alcohol. There was no history of exposure to trauma, toxic materials or recent travel abroad. She was not taking any regular medication and had no known allergies.

The temperature was 36.6°C, the pulse was 72 per minute and the respirations were 14 per minute. The blood pressure was 130/70 mmHg.

On neurological examination, cognitive function, speech and the cranial nerves were normal. Examination of the limbs showed distal symmetrical wasting and weakness in the arms and legs. There was a postural tremor

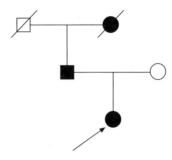

Fig. 29.1. Pedigree of patient's family. In addition to the patient herself, gait disorder and pes cavus were present in her father. Her deceased paternal grandmother had been similarly affected.

of the upper limbs and evidence of sensory ataxia. She was tendon areflexic, plantar responses were unobtainable. Sensory testing revealed impaired position sense to the ankles. Vibration sense was also affected in her feet and in the fingers. She had diminished cutaneous sensation to pinprick, temperature and light touch in a 'glove-and-stocking' distribution, extending to the mid-forearms and to the knees. She was unsteady, without falling, on Rombergs test. Her gait was abnormal with evidence of bilateral foot-drop.

Examination of the cardiovascular and respiratory systems, and the abdomen was normal. General examination was otherwise noncontributory, apart from bilateral pes cavus, and the scars of previous foot surgery.

Routine hematological and biochemical investigations were normal, including full blood count, erythrocyte sedimentation rate, serum urea, electrolytes, calcium, glucose and liver function tests. Thyroid function, syphilis serology, serum vitamin B_{12} and folate were also normal or negative. Serum immunoglobulins were within the normal range, with no paraprotein detected on serum protein electrophoresis. Antinuclear antibodies and rheumatoid factor were negative. Chest X-ray and electrocardiogram were normal. Urinalysis was unremarkable. Cerebrospinal fluid examination showed a protein concentration of 0.7 g/l, with no white cells and normal glucose concentration.

Nerve conduction studies revealed marked slowing of motor nerve conduction velocities to 20 m/s and below in the upper limbs, with prolonged distal motor latencies (8.6 ms for the right median nerve) and absent sensory nerve action potentials. There was evidence of conduction block in the proximal median nerve. The findings were all consistent with a severe demyelinating motor and sensory polyneuropathy.

A diagnostic procedure was performed.

*   *   *

Discussion

This patient's family history (Fig. 29.1) suggests a hereditary basis for her motor and sensory polyneuropathy, with a dominant pattern of inheritance. Genetic causes of polyneuropathy are summarized in Table 29.1, with their modes of inheritance. Of those which are dominant, many may be eliminated immediately. Thus, the familial amyloid polyneuropathies manifest with predominantly sensory and autonomic, or focal, features. The hepatic porphyrias are characterized by recurrent attacks of subacute, mainly motor neuropathy, with associated CNS and gastrointestinal symptoms, triggered by precipitating factors, such as certain drugs, alcohol and intercurrent illness. In the autosomal dominant cerebellar ataxias, neuropathy is usually a relatively minor feature compared to the cerebellar disorder. The only variant of hereditary sensory and autonomic neuropathy with dominant inheritance is type 1. This condition is characterized by sensory loss and tissue injury in the feet. Patients present with callus formation on the soles, painless stress fractures, Charcot arthropathy of the feet and ankles, and recurrent plantar ulcers. Hereditary neuropathy with liability to pressure palsies is a distinctive condition in which peripheral nerves are overly susceptible to mechanical compression or traction. As the name implies, patients present with recurrent, isolated mononeuropathies. Most attacks develop suddenly and recover completely. The disorder is associated with characteristic focal sausage-shaped myelin swellings – *tomacula* – on nerve biopsy.

This leaves only Charcot–Marie–Tooth disease (hereditary motor and sensory neuropathy) as the likely diagnosis. In fact, Charcot–Marie–Tooth disease is a clinically and genetically heterogeneous group of disorders. Their nomenclature is currently evolving, but two main groups are recognized. These are the hypertrophic/demyelinating form (CMT1, also known as hereditary motor and sensory neuropathy (HMSN) type I), and the axonal or, more correctly, neuronal form (CMT2, or HMSN type II).

In CMT1, patients manifest with slowly progressive distal wasting and weakness, the onset often being in childhood. The anterolateral muscle compartment of the leg is particularly affected and bilateral pes cavus, with hammer toes, is found in most patients. Tendon reflexes are usually absent, sensory loss is generally mild. Peripheral nerves are palpably thickened in up to 25% of patients. Electro-diagnostic studies show marked slowing of nerve conduction velocity. There is evidence of segmental demyelination with associated hypertrophy in nerve biopsy specimens. CMT2 resembles CMT1, except that the age of onset may be later. Skeletal deformities are less prominent, peripheral nerves are not enlarged, and nerve conduction velocity is relatively preserved, reflecting the underlying axonal rather than demyelinating pathology. The patient under discussion clearly conforms to CMT1.

Until relatively recently, the subclassification of Charcot–Marie–Tooth disease was limited to the clinical phenotype, supplemented by

Table 29.1. Genetic causes of polyneuropathy.

Disease	Salient features	Inheritance
Charcot–Marie–Tooth	See text	AD/AR/X
Hereditary neuropathy with liability to pressure palsies	See text	AD
Hereditary sensory and autonomic neuropathy	See text	AD/AR
Hereditary motor neuropathy	Synonymous with spinal muscular atrophy	AR (predominantly)
Friedreichs ataxia	Cerebellar and pyramidal signs usually apparent	AR
Spinocerebellar ataxias	See text	AD
Giant axonal neuropathy	Childhood onset, CNS involvement, tightly curled hair	AR
Familial amyloid polyneuropathy	See text	AD
Hepatic porphyrias	See text	AD
Leukodystrophy	Prominent CNS involvement	AR/X
Refsums disease	Phytanic acid storage disease – pigmentary retinopathy, ataxia, neuropathy, deafness, skeletal and skin abnormalities	AR
Fabrys disease	Painful neuropathy, renal failure, vascular disease, skin lesions (angiokeratomas)	X
Abetalipoproteinemia	Acanthocytes, retinitis pigmentosa, neuropathy, ataxia	AR
Tangier disease	Neuropathy with orange tonsils (due to lipid deposition)	AR
Mitochondrial disorders	Neuropathy associated with myopathy and CNS involvement	Mitochondrial

AD = Autosomal dominant; AR = autosomal recessive; X = X-linked.

neurophysiological studies and sometimes nerve biopsy.[1] However, advances in molecular genetics now permit a more exact diagnosis in many cases, based on DNA analysis, which in turn aids genetic counseling. The most common molecular defect associated with CMT1, known as CMT1A, localizes to chromosome 17. Most CMT1A patients have a DNA duplication of a small portion of this chromosome (17p11.2-12).[2] This duplicated region contains the gene for peripheral myelin protein-22 (PMP-22), a membrane glycoprotein apparently involved in myelin compaction. Disease expression relates to a gene dosage effect, caused by three copies of the PMP-22 gene.[3] Interestingly, most patients with hereditary neuropathy with liability to pressure palsies have a deletion of chromosome 17p11.2-12 corresponding to the duplicated region in CMT1A.[4] Again, gene dosage appears to be important, this phenotype resulting from only a single copy of the PMP-22 gene being present. When there are four copies of the gene (homozygous duplication), patients present with a severe, early onset demyelinating neuropathy (CMT3; Dejerine–Sottas disease). A minority of CMT1A patients have point mutations of the PMP-22 gene, rather than the duplication. Other CMT1 patients have a different molecular basis, not involving PMP-22. Thus, for example, CMT1B is associated with point mutations of the P_0 gene on chromosome 1.[5] P_0 is an important adhesion molecule, involved in the formation and compaction of peripheral myelin. Point mutations of the PMP-22 and P_0 genes may also result in the severe CMT3 phenotype. Recently, mutations in yet another gene – the early growth response 2 (EGR-2) gene – have been found in some families with CMT1.[6]

The first diagnostic procedure performed on the patient under discussion was DNA analysis. This confirmed the presence of a duplication of 17p11.2-12, and hence a diagnosis of CMT1A. Despite this clear-cut genetic result, it is noteworthy that the patient deviated in several respects from the typical clinical phenotype. First, she had a postural tremor. However, this is sometimes seen in CMT1 – the *Roussy-Lévy* variant. More importantly, she had more marked sensory features than are usually encountered in CMT1. Paresthesiae, in particular, are much more common in acquired than in inherited neuropathies. Furthermore, she had suffered two episodes of subacute progression of her illness, against a background of much more gradual, chronic deterioration. Finally, her electrophysiological findings were unusual, with the demonstration of conduction block. This is not a regular feature of CMT, though block may be shown at entrapment sites in hereditary neuropathy with liability to pressure palsies. These atypical features prompted a search for a second, superadded cause of polyneuropathy, hence the screening blood and urine tests, which, in the event, proved negative. Her co-existent ulcerative colitis is not likely to be relevant. Various neuropathies have been described in association with this condition, including Guillain–Barré syndrome, autonomic neuropathy, multifocal neuropathy and perineuritis.[7] However, the patient's first subacute episode antedated the onset of the inflammatory bowel disease by 10 years. Furthermore, the second subacute deterioration was not temporally associated with a relapse of colitis.

Because of the continuing uncertainty, the patient underwent a second diagnostic procedure, namely sural nerve fascicular biopsy (Fig. 29.2). This confirmed the typical appearances of CMT1 (Fig. 29.2a). However, inflammatory cell infiltrates were also seen (Fig. 29.2b). This unusual finding, in combination with the atypical clinical features, modestly elevated cerebrospinal fluid protein concentration, and conduction block on nerve conduction studies, suggested the patient had chronic inflammatory demyelinating polyneuropathy in addition to CMT1A. An association between these two conditions has previously been reported.[8] The mechanism by which a subgroup of CMT patients is rendered susceptible to superimposed inflammatory neuropathy, beyond coincidence, is unknown. Immunogenetic studies of associations between chronic inflammatory demyelinating polyneuropathy and specific antigens of the major histocompatibility complex are controversial. Perhaps the extra dose of PMP-22 is relevant, as anti-PMP-22 antibodies have been detected in patients with inflammatory neuropathies.[9]

Treatment of Charcot–Marie–Tooth disease is largely restricted to proper foot care, as illustrated in this patient's case, and genetic counseling. The recognition of the subgroup with a superimposed inflammatory component is potentially important as some of the clinical features may be

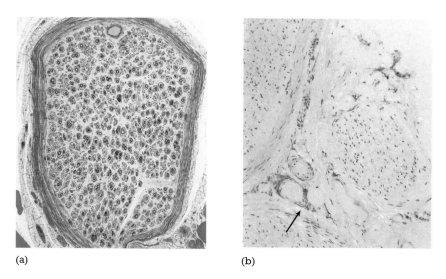

(a)   (b)

Fig. 29.2. Sural nerve fascicular biopsy. (a) Semithin transverse section showing numerous 'onion bulbs' (thionine–acridine orange, ×200). (b) Immunostaining showing epineurial and endoneurial T cell (CD4) infiltrates (arrowed) (×200).

reversible with immunomodulatory treatment. The patient under discussion was treated for her subacute deterioration in hand function with a 5-day course of high-dose intravenous immunoglobulin. She responded, both clinically and electrophysiologically, conduction block no longer being apparent after the therapy.

Diagnosis

Charcot–Marie–Tooth disease (hereditary motor and sensory neuropathy), type 1A, with superadded chronic inflammatory demyelinating polyneuropathy.

References

1. Harding AE, Thomas PK. The clinical features of hereditary motor and sensory neuropathy types I and II. *Brain* 1980; **103**: 259–280.
2. Lupski JR, deOca-Luna RM, Slaugenhaupt S et al. DNA duplication associated with Charcot–Marie–Tooth disease type 1A. *Cell* 1991; **66**: 219–232.
3. Gabriel JM, Erne B, Pareyson D et al. Gene dosage effect in hereditary peripheral neuropathy. Expression of peripheral myelin protein 22 in Charcot–Marie–Tooth disease type 1A and hereditary neuropathy with liability to pressure palsies nerve biopsies. *Neurology* 1997; **49**: 1635–1640.
4. Chance PF, Alderson MK, Leppig KA et al. DNA deletion associated with hereditary neuropathy with liability to pressure palsies. *Cell* 1993; **72:** 143–151.
5. Hayasaka K, Himoro M, Sato W et al. Charcot–Marie–Tooth neuropathy type 1B is associated with mutations of the myelin P_0 gene. *Nat Genet* 1993; **5**: 31–34.
6. Warner LE, Mancias P, Butler IJ et al. Mutations in the early growth response 2 (EGR-2) gene are associated with hereditary myelinopathies. *Nat Genet* 1998; **18**: 382–384.
7. Chad DA, Smith TW, DeGirolami U, Hammer K. Perineuritis and ulcerative colitis. *Neurology* 1986; **36**: 1377–1379.
8. Dyck PJ, Swanson CJ, Low PA et al. Prednisone-responsive hereditary motor and sensory neuropathy. *Mayo Clin Proc* 1982; **57**: 239–246.
9. Gabriel CM, Gregson NA, Hughes RAC. Anti-PMP22 antibodies in patients with inflammatory neuropathy. *J Neuroimmunol* 2000; **104**: 139–146.

List of cases, authors and final diagnosis

Index